T0133907

Higher Professional Education for General Practitioners

Ed Peile FRCP FRCGP MRCPCH
Associate Adviser, Oxford Deanery
Associate Director of Clinical Studies, University of Oxford

Glynis Buckle MSc Cert Med Ed ILT(M)
HPE Tutor, Oxford Deanery
CPD Tutor, Leicestershire, Northamptonshire and Rutland Deanery

and

Derek Gallen FRCGP MEd ILT(M)
Director of Postgraduate General Practice Education
Oxford Deanery

Foreword by

Professor Arthur Hibble

Radcliffe Medical Press

Radcliffe Medical Press Ltd
18 Marcham Road
Abingdon
Oxon OX14 1AA
United Kingdom

www.radcliffe-oxford.com
The Radcliffe Medical Press electronic catalogue and online ordering
facility.
Direct sales to anywhere in the world.

British Library Cataloguing in Publication Data

A catalogue record for this book is available from the British Library.

ISBN 1 85775 968 0

Typeset by Advance Typesetting Ltd, Oxfordshire
Printed and bound by TJ International Ltd, Padstow, Cornwall

Contents

Foreword

If medical education has a holy grail then it must be the continuum. Years of striving, acres of print and hours of discussion have only succeeded in defining the transitions.

The HPE movement grew out of a realisation that the three years of vocational training for general practice were not an adequate preparation for GP principalship. The background is recorded in this book. If this narrative describes the conception and gestation, then the birth was managed through the first two Cambridge Conferences.

Several important principles were defined. Amongst these were that HPE is a case study within continuing professional development, the transitions are a necessary element of professional development and that they can be managed well or badly. The case for HPE needed to be made in educational and political terms; and out of the many possible names 'Higher Professional Education' was felt to be the most appropriate. It is, of course, inevitable that other countries have subsequently used the term differently. The Dutch, for instance, use HPE to define the further education undertaken by established practitioners to do what we in the UK would describe as a 'GP with a Special Interest'.

This book describes both the transitions and the curriculum and, through the case study that is HPE, offers theoretically argued practical solutions. In so doing it offers clinical educators a rationale for curriculum building in any and all of the phases of professional development. This is not just a book for HPE programme directors or tutors, nor do its conclusions confine it to UK practice.

As such, it also adds to the growing, powerful arguments for the professionalisation of medical education. Educational supervision in medicine requires the same depth of knowledge and skills as does doctoring. This theoretical base manifests itself in the praxis of defining learning needs, delivering the solutions and making the assessments.

The future of HPE as a distinct phase in UK GP education will need to be argued as it seeks to move from development to establishment. Several tests will be applied by the funders and the educators. These must include – how is the transition between supervised and autonomous practice managed?, and – does the young professional have a sustainable way of defining her continuing personal professional development within the context of practice? In short, are the educational programmes delivering GPs fit for today's and tomorrow's health service? Only the active practitioners can provide the answers through critical reflective action research, and this book offers a clear framework from which to derive the questions that will deliver the answers.

Professor Arthur Hibble
Director of Postgraduate General Practice Education
Eastern Deanery PGMDE
Cambridge
May 2003

Preface

Continuing professional development is a concept that doctors still struggle to comprehend and introduce into their professional lives. All too often we see our education split into discrete entities like passing finals, passing summative assessment and undertaking 30 hours of education each year to obtain our postgraduate education allowance. The concept that medical education is a continuum from entering medical school through to retirement needs to be embraced if we are to make full use of the opportunities available to us by finding the right time to improve our knowledge and skills. This improvement could then be reflected in better care for our patients.

There is a need for individual doctors to have an overview of the educational opportunities that are available when they are in training and when they have qualified. This would also allow those who plan educational provision to target the needs of the profession more specifically, and to produce doctors 'fit for purpose'.

The introduction of higher professional education (HPE) is a great asset in delivering better-qualified GPs at a time when many feel ill-equipped for partnerships. Newly qualified GPs often seek work as a non-principal because they feel too inexperienced for partnership or because their domestic situation prevents them from settling in a particular area.

Although vocational training has been seen as an end-point of training we know that it is just the start of continuing professional development. HPE enables newly qualified doctors to focus on areas in which they still feel unsure or need more training. It enables those planning vocational training schemes to acknowledge the impact and place of the period of

HPE. It can therefore relieve some of the obvious pressures on an already full vocational training curriculum.

In this book we have sought to outline the issues concerning the introduction of HPE. We hope to engage readers in reflecting on their own past experiences and planning their future educational needs. This book should help those who are currently undertaking HPE and those that are responsible for the delivery of educational programmes for those in their first year post-vocational training scheme. Above all we hope readers enjoy this book and embrace the opportunities presented in HPE to become life-long learners.

Ed Peile
Glynis Buckle
Derek Gallen
May 2003

About the authors

Dr Ed Peile leads on Higher Professional Education for Oxford Deanery, where he is an Associate Adviser. Ed started a single-handed practice in 1983 and began GP Registrar training in 1986. He still contributes to the teaching at Aston Clinton Surgery, which is now part of a larger PMS grouping, focused on education from undergraduates to GP Retainers. Since 1998, Ed has been at the University of Oxford, where he has been undertaking Doctoral studies on process and outcome in GP Registrar education. Ed directs the Oxford Deanery New Teachers' Course, and has responsibilities for faculty development. Ed's interests in medical education include appraisal and interprofessional education. He is an elected Board Member at CAIPE and an Editorial Adviser on medical education to the *BMJ*.

Glynis Buckle has been a practice manager since 1989 and still has an active role in her Northamptonshire practice. She became a Continuing Professional Development (CPD) Tutor in 2001 and a Clinical Tutor in General Practice in 2003. She is also a tutor on the Oxford Deanery New Teachers' Course. Glynis has co-authored four books on primary care management and personal and practice development plans. Her particular areas of interest are in interprofessional learning and organisational development.

Dr Derek Gallen is the Director of Postgraduate General Practice Education for the Oxford Deanery. He was appointed as a trainer in 1993 and a GP tutor in 1996. He then became the associate adviser for Northamptonshire in 1999 and then

Director in 2001. Derek's interest in medical education include educational needs assessment and interprofessional learning. He has written three books on topics related to starting in practice, primary care management and personal and practice development plans. He is editorial adviser to *Update* magazine and *Doctor* newspaper and still does one day a week in general practice.

Acknowledgements

We particularly wish to acknowledge the following people:

- Dr Regina Conradt for her collation and interpretation of data.
- Gillian Nineham (Radcliffe Medical Press) for her support throughout the process.
- Verna Kitchener, our very accomplished and very understanding PA.
- Marion Lynch, Honor Merriman and Bren Sainsbury who make up the Oxford Deanery HPE team.

To Linda for putting up with my struggles to work on the book at the same time as everything else.

Ed

To Noel for all the TLC.

Glynis

To my family for their continued support.

Derek

1

An introduction to higher professional education (HPE)

Higher professional education (HPE) was introduced in October 2001 in response to requests from the profession to cater for the needs of newly qualified general practitioners (GPs). In essence, HPE is the provision of 20 days of education, with locum costs, and a small contribution to course fees. It is applicable in the first year after a doctor has finished the vocational training scheme. The profession had clearly hoped that funding would be for 20 days per year for the first two years after vocational training, but has had to accept a pragmatic solution in the current economic climate.

HPE is not a criticism of the gaps that vocational training has failed to cover. Indeed, one of the successes of vocational training is the breadth and scope of the education offered. HPE should be seen as a further opportunity for individuals to develop skills and knowledge while actually undertaking the role of GPs. The curriculum to develop a doctor 'fit for purpose' will change over time. We need to look at the relationship between undergraduate learning, pre-registration house jobs, vocational training and HPE to grasp whether at each stage we have a doctor 'fit for purpose'. In this model, HPE will free up time on vocational training schemes as the curriculum is honed to look at the specific achievable knowledge, skills and attitudes pertinent to the three-year programme.

Vocational training

The current arrangements of vocational training for general practice in the UK were developed in the late 1960s and early 1970s. They became embodied in the vocational training regulations (NHS, England and Wales, 1979) that have been mandatory for entering practice as a principal within the British National Health Service (NHS) since 1982. The purpose of vocational training for general practice is to give doctors in the UK skills, the knowledge and competencies necessary to work in general practice and meet the needs of NHS patients. The vocational training regulations that were passed by an act of Parliament in 1976 stipulated only a three-year training programme.

Many question whether a standard vocational training scheme of only three years' duration is long enough. Are doctors ready for a lifetime of practice at completion of their vocational training scheme? The Royal College of General Practitioners (RCGP) did not think so when vocational training schemes were about to be introduced. The RCGP argued for a five-year scheme, which would have put GPs more on a level with their specialist trainee colleagues (RCGP, 1996). Giving evidence to a Royal Commission on Education in 1996, the College considered the options for 'Senior Registrars' and other ways of extending the learning experience of young doctors. It was not alone in considering three years too short, and already government thinking was moving this way (Calman, 1998). Experience from around the country was that vocational training could not possibly meet all the young doctors' needs in practice (Bonsor *et al.*, 1998). However, the vocational training scheme has remained a three-year programme, of which 18 months may be taken in general practice. In reality, because of funding implications and the need for service provision in hospitals, 12 rather than 18 months has become the normal time spent in general practice, with the remaining two years spent in hospital.

More recently, however, many innovative vocational training schemes have developed throughout the country to include 18 months in general practice. The availability of such schemes has served to increase the job satisfaction of those GP registrars who are able to access them (Lawrence, 2000).

Although HPE was introduced to help bridge and fill some of the gaps left by vocational training schemes in the development of competent GPs, we should not forget the benefits and learning opportunities that are available within vocational training. The impossibility of encompassing the whole of general practice learning within vocational training has been well documented and the problems are outlined in Chapter 3. However, whereas we quite rightly look to see how vocational training could be improved, we often fail to consider its good points and the areas that have real value in the development of future GPs.

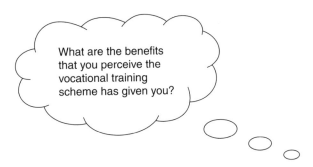

What are the benefits that you perceive the vocational training scheme has given you?

The vast majority of doctors qualifying as GPs have joined formal training schemes. This is clearly not the only route to becoming a GP as many other doctors have made up their own scheme in order to fulfil the Joint Committee on Postgraduate Training for General Practice (JCPTGP) regulations. The great advantage of joining a formal training scheme is that it provides job security for three years. Many training schemes also have the day release course running during the hospital component, though clearly in some jobs and some specialities this becomes difficult at times due to service provision. There is evidence that vocationally trained GPs are better doctors in terms of performing the task of a GP to a level of providing quality care (Hindmarsh *et al.*, 1998).

During general practice training, doctors will learn and work in a variety of hospitals and general practices. They can do a variety of jobs and have very different work experiences, depending on the locality and the resources of the vocational training schemes (Baker, 1993). The hospital phase of training is an important part of the postgraduate training of general practice. Suitable hospital posts offer training GPs the opportunity to allocate time for more detailed investigation and more sophisticated management of many illnesses than may be possible in general practice within a more concentrated and time-limited environment. The training builds on experience gained in the pre-registration period and enables doctors to acquire increasing responsibility for the care of patients as they gather experience and become confident under the supervision of the hospital educational supervisor (DoH, 2000). The common specialities are:

*   general medicine
*   geriatric medicine
*   paediatrics
*   psychiatry

with one of:

*   accident and emergency
*   or general surgery
*   or accident and emergency medicine with either general surgery or orthopaedic surgery

with one of:

*   obstetrics
*   gynaecology
*   or obstetrics and gynaecology.

These may be approved for general practice training by the JCPTGP.

It is also possible to obtain prescribed experience by completing a maximum of six months in other hospital jobs relevant to general practice. More and more schemes in the country are looking to these opportunities, not only to improve the diversity of training options but to expand their schemes to recruit more doctors to general practice. Combinations of posts are favoured by the registrars, for example dermatology, ENT and ophthalmology; however, they are less favoured by the trusts. This is because registrars, moving from the job after, say, three months in post, are perceived to have been trained but not to have had enough time to offer a full service commitment commensurate with the training. This is a difficult point for some hospital posts but the reality is that the senior house officers (SHOs) are training grades (Baker, 1993).

The new proposals for the reform of the SHO grade (Donaldson, 2002) have far-reaching implications for the development and education of this group of doctors. Since half of all doctors in training are in this grade, any changes will have a 'knock-on' effect to other hospital grades and other health professionals.

There are five key principles as outlined in the consultation document to reform the SHO grade (Donaldson, 2002).

1   Training should be programme-based.
2   Training should begin with broadly based programmes pursued by all trainees.
3   Programmes should be time-limited.
4   Training should allow for individually tailored or personal programmes.
5   Arrangements should facilitate movement into and out of training and between training programmes.

Although the exact details of the delivery of the programmes are not yet finalised, it is suggested that there would be a foundation programme and a basic specialist training programme.

In the two-year foundation programme, the first year would be similar to the current pre-registration year. The second year would build on the first, with more of the generic skills essential to all doctors (for example, communication skills). This would then be followed by the basic specialist training programme (Donaldson, 2002).

The implications for general practice training derive from the fact that the minimum period of vocational training is, by statute, currently three years. In order to meet this criterion individuals could spend some part of the second foundation year in general practice followed by a two-year general practice programme that incorporated practice and hospital posts similar to the current system. This should bring into sharp relief the roles of hospital posts in the delivery of a future general practice workforce. It would not be acceptable to have educational teaching that focused on those doctors who were specialising in the subject. More primary care-focused teaching is needed and that may mean that general practice trainers or course organisers would become more involved in the hospital teaching of GP registrars.

GP registrars are dissatisfied with many aspects of the training within the hospital setting but many of these areas of dissatisfaction, for example, informal teaching, inadequate feedback, problems with study leave and difficulty attending the general practice day release, are all slowly but surely being sorted out. Evans (2002) suggests that

'Postgraduate general practice training in hospital-based posts was seen as poor quality, irrelevant and run as if it were of secondary importance to service commitments. In contrast, general practice-based postgraduate training was widely praised for good formal teaching that met educational needs.' (Evans, 2002, pp. 1–33)

Hospital trainees now have:

- a named educational supervisor
- personal education objectives

- logbooks
- formal assessment
- feedback on performance and
- feedback to departments.

(STA, 2003)

This named educational supervisor, as a mentor, can mirror the same process that registrars undergo with their trainers in general practice in the registrar year. The inclusion of educational objectives within any of the hospital components is a welcome addition, allowing doctors to be in a much better position to identify what they can learn from their day-to-day work. These objectives are now put into logbooks, which in reality are becoming the precursors to the personal development plans that all GPs need to have in the future (Paice *et al.*, 1997; Gallen and Buckle, 2001). The use and content of these logbooks are essential during the formal appraisal, which occurs half way through the post and should also occur at the end of each post.

Feedback on performance is important for learners. This is an area in which trainers are increasingly becoming involved, in conjunction with hospital consultants, to ensure that not only does the appraisal process take place but that there is suitable emphasis placed on general practice elements of hospital specialities. Hand's (2000) paper on satisfaction with hospital training for general practice showed an increase in satisfaction with the induction process for all the SHO posts from 1996 to 1999. There was also an increase in the number of SHOs who would recommend that post to a friend. It is clear from this work that there is still a long way to go to ensure that hospital posts are meeting not only individuals' perceived requirements within the speciality but also the requirements for producing GPs fit for the future. The proposed reforms for the SHO grade may well go some way to addressing the balance between the generic skills needed by all doctors in order to practise medicine and integration into specialist training, of which general practice plays a key role.

HPE fits very well into this new model as it recognises that education does not stop at the end of the prescribed training programme but continues through life-long learning. The period of HPE following the vocational training scheme enables doctors to look at personal educational needs within the context of the working environment. It is therefore timely that HPE has been introduced and focuses on the educational needs of individuals in their particular work environment and can go some way to addressing many of the issues raised.

HPE: an answer to a problem?

Education is an investment for individuals and governments alike. When HPE was introduced, the NHS had to find new money to fund not only the educational provision but also the clinical replacement time.

Here are a few of the reasons why certain stakeholders might see it as worthwhile to invest in HPE. Take a moment to fill in Table 1.1 with + or ++ or +++, depending on how strongly you rate the motivation to invest for each of the three groups.

Table 1.1:   Major stakeholders in HPE: what are they concerned about?

Issue	Government/ Society	Partners/ Colleagues	Individual doctor
Retention of scarce doctors			
Recruitment			
Improved patient safety			
Enhanced clinical performance			
Managerial contribution			
Professional satisfaction			
Embedding life-long learning patterns			
Reducing pressure on vocational training scheme			

What did you see as the driving forces behind the government's investment? We think it was all those reasons but retention, recruitment and safety are likely to have been the levers that released treasury funds, with professional satisfaction a desirable outcome.

HPE: is it really new?

For many years around the country doctors newly in practice have been getting together in formal or informal groupings to extend their learning and to support each other through the difficult early years as a GP (Plant, 1993; Smith, 2001). Sometimes these groups took particular formats, such as some of the Balint groups (Marinker, 1970; Samuel, 1989). Other processes were being developed simultaneously to support young doctors, including mentoring (Freeman, 1998). Mohanna (1999), from Staffordshire, looked at what made a successful young principals' group and reported nine key points, including the observation that to obtain maximum benefits, individuals should attend a mixture of task, process and group dynamics resulting in the development of leadership skills. Earlier, Baron and Evans (1998) surveyed young principals. These authors found that many felt unprepared in their early days as a GP. Baron and Evans (1998) identified partnerships, clinical knowledge gaps, practice and personal management as many of the issues and these topics have influenced the agenda for many young principals' groups.

In some parts of the country more systematic attempts to develop relevant learning were underway (Pitts *et al.*, 1999; Baron and Evans, 1998). In name as well as in concept, these schemes were paving the way for HPE as we know it today. Two national conferences hosted by the Anglia region raised the profile of these schemes and undoubtedly influenced the decision of government to formally introduce HPE (Hibble, 1996, 1998).

References

Baker M (1993) Enhancing the educational content of SHO posts. *British Medical Journal* **306**, 808–809.

Baron R and Evans R (1998) The training needs of young principals. *Education for General Practice* **9**, 403–409.

Bonsor R, Gibbs T and Woodward R (1998) Vocational training and beyond – listening to voices from a void. *British Journal of General Practice* **48**, 915–918.

Calman K (1998) *A Review of Continuing Professional Development in General Practice.* DoH, London.

Department of Health (2000) *The GP Registrar Scheme. Vocational Training for General Medical Practice. The UK Guide.* DoH, London.

Donaldson L (2002) *Unfinished Business. Proposals for Reform of the Senior House Officer Grade.* DoH, London.

Evans J, Lambert T *et al.* (2002) *GP Recruitment and Retention: a qualitative analysis of doctors' comments about training for and working in general practice.* Occasional Paper No. 83, pp. 1–33. Royal College of General Practitioners, London.

Freeman R (1998) *Mentoring in General Practice.* Butterworth Heinemann, Oxford.

Gallen D and Buckle G (2001) *Personal and Practice Development Plans in Primary Care.* Butterworth Heinemann, Oxford.

Hand C (2000) Evaluating satisfaction with hospital training for general practice: a comparison of two surveys in East Anglia for the JCPTGP using the RCGP SHO questionnaire. *Education for General Practice* **11**, 385–390.

Hibble A (1996) *Report of the First Cambridge Conference on Higher Professional Education for General Practice.* Cambridge, Anglia Region.

Hibble A (1998) *Report of the Second Cambridge Conference on Higher Professional Education for General Practice.* Cambridge, Anglia Region.

Hindmarsh JH, Coster GD and Gilbert C (1998) Are vocational trained general practitioners better GPs? A review of research designs and outcomes. *Medical Educators* **32**, 244–254.

Lawrence DK (2000) Extended general practice training. *Education for General Practice* **11**, 1–24.

Marinker M (1970) Balint seminars and vocational training in general practice. *Journal of the Royal College of General Practitioners* **19**, 79–91.

Mohanna K (1999) Bridging the gap. What makes a successful young principals' group? *Education for General Practice* **10**, 245–251.

National Health Service (NHS) England and Wales (1979) *The National Health Service (Vocational Training) Regulations. No. 1644.* HMSO, London.

Paice E, Moss F, West G and Grant J (1997) Association of a log book and experience as a pre-registration home officer: interview survey. *British Medical Journal* **314**, 213–216.

Pitts J, Curtis A, While R and Holloway I (1999) Practice professional development plans: general practitioners' perspectives on proposed changes in general practice education. *British Journal of General Practice* **49**, 959–962.

Plant G (1993) Young principals and their problems. *Postgraduate Education for General Practice* **4**, 184–191.

Royal College of General Practitioners (1996) *Evidence to the Royal Commission on Medical Education.* RCGP, London.

Samuel O (1989) How doctors learn in a Balint group. *Family Practice* **6**, 108–113.

Smith L and Wright T (2001) Expectations and benefits of the Somerset New Principals Course: ten years of experience in one year. *Education for General Practice* **12**, 169–177.

Specialist Training Authority (2003) *Policy Statement: Supervision of Trainees.* www.sta-mrc.org.uk/supervision_of_trainees.html (accessed 10/4/03).

2

What do trainers offer that has lasting value?

Introduction

There seems little doubt that all doctors completing their vocational training schemes, and embarking on a career in general practice, have numerous educational needs to meet in the course of their professional practice (Gallen and Buckle, 2001). Before examining how best to do this in the early years after certification, it is helpful to think about the process of the education that immediately precedes it: how can the long-term benefit of vocational training be maximised? Education is a continuum: from medical school through house and SHO posts to the GP registrar year, perhaps extended by enhanced training, and on to HPE and the world of continuing professional development in practice.

The context of HPE is the vocational training which precedes it, and the professional practice which continues afterwards. In this chapter we will explore what aspects of vocational training have had lasting value for practitioners, and consider the implications for HPE.

A research project seeking the views of former vocational training scheme registrars

Aylesbury Vocational Training Scheme is one of eight schemes in the Oxford Postgraduate Deanery. At a residential training session, the current trainers bemoaned the lack of evidence on how trainers are 'adding value' to their trainees' learning process (Crawley and Levin, 1990; Hindmarsh *et al.*, 1998). This led eventually to an NHS R&D funded initiative to look at how the process of training affects practitioner quality.

The project started with the researcher interviewing as many former registrars as possible, to ascertain their views. The ensuing research project has been described elsewhere (Peile *et al.*, 2001) and resulted in the delineation of categories of educational behaviours in general practice education, each with a dimension which spanned behaviour between – at one end – behaviour deemed to be helpful in the long-term and – at the other – behaviour which was unhelpful. All the categories selected have been meaningful to audiences of GP trainers, educators and current registrars, providing evidence of face validity.

> What has been of lasting value to you from your vocational training? What approaches and educational behaviours did you find helpful?

What helped vocational training scheme-trained doctors?

The categories and dimensions are summarised in Table 2.1, but each individual category will be explored in more detail shortly.

Table 2.1:   The categories and dimensions summarised

1	Training or education	**Problem-based approach** Teaching based on approaches to problems which are not limited to present-day contexts	**Emphasis on managing disease** Teaching focused on current policies for disease management
2	Style spectrum	**Wide variety of styles** Learner exposed to different consulting styles and role-models in tutorials	**Narrow range of styles** Teaching dominated by personal style and behaviour of trainer
3	Space for reflection	**Encouraging reflective practitioner** Safe environment to learn from mistakes	**Protocol-driven behaviour** Black and white approach adopted where learner is expected to adhere to guidelines and elements of blame culture likely
4	Modelling personal development and team skills	**Personal development and team management skills taught** Guided learning of skills such as time management, assertiveness, boundary-setting	**No emphasis on team behaviours** Little attempt is made to help learner understand the importance of team-working and the areas of personal development that are involved
5	Learning cycles	**Learning cycles completed** A culture exists in the practice where reflection, audit, assessment all promote change and re-evaluation	**Haphazard change** Culture is reactive to external pressures, and little evidence of information about the practice inspiring meaningful change
6	Family practice in context	**Contextualised learning** Trainer introduces the broader dimensions of family and health expectations	**Emphasis on presenting problem** Focus remains on sorting and shifting
7	Control and direction	**Learner-centred approach** Trainer listens to trainee and positively seeks out their educational needs, adapting the training accordingly	**Trainer-centred approach** Trainer adopts rigid structure with fixed views on the educational diet to feed trainees
8	Feedback	**Sensitive feedback** Both positive and negative feedback delivered where appropriate, stimulating confidence in the learner, and encouraging change	**Inappropriate criticism** Feedback either inadequate or misplaced or poorly delivered, often not timely or specific enough to be useful to learner

Can educational behaviours be assessed in training practices?

In the second phase of research, we wanted to assess how trainers manifest these behaviours. In order not to overburden the training practices, an approach to assessing these behaviours by use of mainly the same techniques that are already employed on re-accreditation visits was piloted.

Re-accreditation visits

Training practices all currently undergo educational assessment for the purposes of accreditation and re-accreditation. The crux of each assessment is a peer-review visit. Over the past 20 years, in Oxford these have been made to all trainers, at a minimum of four-yearly intervals, by teams of two GP training peers and a team leader (Schofield and Hasler, 1984a, 1984b, 1984c). Since 1992, teams have also included a practice manager from a training practice, who has contributed to the assessment of practice organisation in the visited training practice (Johnson *et al.*, 1997). The criteria for approval and re-approval of training practices have been revised over the years, and criteria and visit schedules have been aligned with national recommendations (JCGPT, 2001).

Agenda for Oxford Deanery visits to training practices

The agenda for the visit always includes the following components.

- Personal interview with practice manager by visiting practice manager.*
- Group or personal interviews with all other administration staff by visiting practice manager.

- Personal interview with each trainer by all visitors together.*
- Group interviews with all members of nursing teams by visitors, singly or in groups.
- Personal interview with current GP registrar in post by all visitors together.*
- Group interview with other doctors by all visitors.
- Inspection of all records of training (logbooks and programme).*
- Inspection of library and online learning resources.
- Inspection of audits, protocols and guidelines.*
- Visiting doctors review a videotape of each trainer consulting.
- Visiting doctors review a videotape of the trainer in tutorial with the GP registrar.*

Items marked with an asterisk are those which prove particularly useful for collecting evidence about training behaviours.

After the visit, team leaders prepare a report, which forms the basis of the decision by the Appointments Committee to accredit or re-accredit a trainer or training practice. Over the course of one year, the extent to which committee decisions under the present system reliably reflected impressions of the visiting team on the quality of the training that a GP registrar would currently receive was evaluated (Peile *et al.*, 2001).

Team leaders have bi-annual training days at which the conduct of the visits is reviewed. At one of these sessions, a wish to increase the emphasis on the *process* of the educational activity was expressed, and research appeared to reflect this, so team leaders were keen to include an assessment of training behaviours on the practice visits.

A training pack was designed to train teams in the somewhat complex process of collecting relevant pieces of evidence about the educational process in the practice (Figure 2.1).

In our pilot work testing opportunities for assessing training behaviours on training visits, a 'standard scenario' was included (*see* Box 2.1). This was designed to pose common educational

Category 1: Training or education

Problem-based approach *Teaching based on approaches to problems which are not limited to present-day contexts (preferred behaviour)*			**Emphasis on managing disease** *Teaching focused on current policies for disease management (less helpful behaviour)*	
Very strong **5**	**Strong** **4**	**Intermediate/neutral** **3**	**Fairly weak** **2**	**Very weak** **1**
	(T) Eating disorders and issues around			
	(V) Prompting for general issues		(R) He expects me to know how to manage things from just reading protocols	
(V) Breast lump mismanagement turned to 'How do I deal with things I know nothing about?'				

Category 2: Style spectrum

Wide variety of styles *Learner exposed to different consulting styles and role-models in tutorials (preferred behaviour)*			**Narrow range of styles** *Teaching dominated by personal style and behaviour of trainer (less helpful behaviour)*	
Very strong **5**	**Strong** **4**	**Intermediate/neutral** **3**	**Fairly weak** **2**	**Very weak** **1**
		(L) Not adventurous use of other team members in tutorial plans		
(R) Everybody is involved in teaching me and I learn from all			(R) He wants me to model myself on him	
			(T) I ask the others to teach on specific subjects *(rather than letting them choose)*	
		(SS) No mention of involving other members		

Figure 2.1: Extract from training pack: composite illustration of evidence recording Category 1: training or education – and Category 2: Style spectrum. Key to evidence sources: T = trainer interview; R = registrar interview; V = video of tutorial; L = logbooks and records of training; SS = standard scenario.

Box 2.1:   Standard scenario

Your registrar is nine months into the training year. She catches you after morning surgery with a problem she wants help sorting out. She has just seen a 24-year-old woman, who is significantly unhappy about her large breasts and wants surgery (reduction mammoplasty), which she cannot afford privately. The consultation has revealed that the patient's breasts have contributed to her low self-image, which has been evident over past years, and may well have played a part in a depressive episode last year (following a relationship breakdown), as well as contributing to aching shoulders. The registrar is aware that cosmetic surgery is classed as a 'Low priority procedure' for referral purposes. This means that she would have to make a special case, and she has promised to ring the patient back after discussing the matter with you, the trainer.

Problem posed – the registrar, conscious of a responsibility to husband resources, wants to know if she should refer the patient to secondary care.

Try to describe in detail how you would handle this question, and where it might lead.

....

Answer guide

Preferred responses
- Asking the registrar to elicit the advantages and disadvantages of agreeing to the patient's request. (**Space for reflection**)
- Referring to guidelines *after* learner has had a chance to think out a strategy in her own way (that is, as a reference for checking out how her treatment plan fits in with conventional advice). (**Space for reflection**)
- A strategy which involves the registrar in thinking about the educational issues raised and how she might address them. (**Control and direction**)
- Constructing an *approach* to the problem which has wider relevance than just sorting the case in question. (**Training or education**)
- Checking that *context* is considered in responding – rather than producing one answer for all women with large breasts. (**Family practice in context**)

Unhelpful behaviours

- Referring learner straight to authority, for example '*Look at the practice protocol*' or '*Ring up Public Health*'. (**Space for reflection**)

- Didactic advice on what to do. (**Space for reflection**)

- Limiting response to this specific case without attempting to guide learning of a generaliseable nature. (**Training or education**)

- Considering the referral issue in isolation (for example, getting hung up on whether reduction mammoplasty is cosmetic surgery). (**Family practice in context**)

Other behaviours such as feedback may be demonstrated in the trainer's response.

problems encountered by trainees in a format which tested trainers' style of response to learners' questions. Answer guides were written, describing examples of possible responses, designating 'preferred behaviour' in different categories and alternative responses indicating 'less helpful behaviour'.

This assessment is similar to the use of standard patient scenarios in the clinical assessment of GPs (Rethans and Saebu, 1977). Although standard scenarios had proved very useful on pilot visits, team leaders rejected them as impractical, and perhaps too open to 'practised responses' on the part of trainers.

We now have one year's experience of teams attempting to incorporate assessment of educational behaviours into their visits, by use of the methods illustrated in Table 2.2. Note that these methods are all using standard components of the visit, outlined in the visit agenda above.

It has proved possible to collect relevant information on all eight categories of training behaviours. It remains to be seen if all these categories will prove useful in formative or summative assessment of GP trainers. At least we will have information on how trainers perform in each category, which will help to shed light on where to place the emphasis in continuing education of trainers.

Table 2.2: Examples of opportunities for assessing training behaviours on re-accreditation visits to training practices

	Category
Training log and programme	
Is the emphasis (after first month) more on managing disease or developing a problem-based approach?	1
Is there broad exposure of learner to other doctors and team members through year?	2
What are the opportunities in the programme for personal development learning about self and teams?	4
Is learning about audit programmed into timetable?	5
Does log reveal evidence of encouragement towards self-direction?	7
Is trainer feedback recorded and tracked?	8
Registrar interview	
Emphasis in teaching on managing disease, or problem-based approach?	1
Good exposure to other doctors and team members all year?	2
Reflective practice encouraged and facilitated?	3
Opportunities found for learning about self and teams?	4
Has learner seen tangible change happen as result of previous audit projects in the practice?	5
Does learner understand educational needs assessment?	5
Does team encourage contextual thinking about family practice?	6
Is there evidence of trainer having encouraged appropriate learner self-direction?	7
Comfortable feedback received? Can learner give examples of positive and negative feedback received?	8

Continued overleaf

Table 2.2:   Continued

	Category
Video of tutorial	
Is the emphasis didactic on managing disease or Socratic, developing a problem-based approach?	1
Is reflective practice modelled and encouraged?	3
Are opportunities used for learning about self and teams?	4
Is there evidence of family contextualisation?	6
Is there ad hoc evidence of trainer adapting to learner stage?	7
Is sensitive feedback demonstrated?	8
Trainer interview	
Does trainer emphasise need to learn disease management protocols or adopt more of a problem-based approach to teaching?	1
How is reflective practice encouraged?	2
What opportunities has trainer offered for learning about self and teams?	4
Is needs assessment modelled as a part of care process?	5
Is needs assessment a part of educational process?	5
What evidence can trainer offer of encouraging appropriate learner self-direction?	7
Is trainer comfortable giving feedback? Give examples of positive and negative feedback	8
Records of training	
Does development of learner's project reveal evidence of understanding importance of completing audit cycle?	5
Do the protocols and guidelines encourage reflective practice or are they didactic?	3

Category numbers refer to the categories of training behaviours defined in Table 2.1.

We also found it helpful, in individual feedback to trainers, to have evidence of their performance across the wide variety of categories. No trainer performed uniformly 'well' across all categories, so we were able to offer evidence of relative strengths and weakness to each trainer and suggest areas for possible improvement, as well as selecting areas for commendation.

Quality descriptors in professional education

To describe a behaviour as *good* or *bad*, *better* or *worse*, *improvable* or *commendable*, is to suggest that we have established that our descriptors of 'preferred behaviour' and 'less helpful behaviour' have some established validity. As yet they do not. They rest on *perceptions* which have yet to be validated by the final phase of this project. However, we subscribe to the pragmatism that underpins action research paradigms, and we feel that we should not wait for 'proof' of benefit before working with research findings to improve practice.

If what is offered to trainers as evidence of their training behaviours has face validity to them as practitioners, and if this evidence suggests change which seems to them productive and beneficial, they are likely to change in that direction.

A technical problem we encountered was the difficulty of making a cross-sectional assessment of a longitudinal process. GP trainers work with registrars over a whole year, and this period often sees progression in craft learners from being 'dependent learners' towards becoming 'self-directed learners'. The work of Grow (1991) suggests that it is helpful if the teaching style matches the need of the learner, changing along an axis between 'authority, expert' to 'delegator' (Grow, 1991).

This is especially important when considering Category 1: 'Training or education', as the needs of novices are different from the needs of advanced practitioners in this respect. The former, in say the first month or two, need more of the somewhat didactic behaviour, labelled as 'less helpful', in order to become proficient. Once they have learnt some of the tools of the trade, the needs of registrars change towards the more Socratic behaviours, labelled as 'preferred', for the bulk of their time in the training practice.

Judicious use of scenarios depicting learners at different stages of training (from the one available for interview to the one taking part in the video tutorial) may show evidence of how trainers adapt to different circumstances, and may provide better evidence of what trainers probably *do*, rather than the evidence of what they *say* they do. Questions such as, 'How do you adapt your training style for learners at different stages?' tend to attract rather hypothetical answers.

Reflecting on ethics in medical education

When a medical school decides to change part of the curriculum, or the way in which students are assessed, it is not common practice to seek ethics committee consent to evaluate the educational changes. Similarly here, the decision was taken by the Deanery to incorporate new assessments of teaching behaviours into assessment visits, and to research the value of these. Should we have sought ethics consent? What are the precepts to guide us in research on medical education?

Ultimately, much of the justification of this work depends on whether it can be shown that certain training behaviours improve the quality of performance of trained practitioners, and whether assessing these behaviours leads to positive change in trainers' performance. Time will tell!

In taking a more detailed look at the categories, we quote extensively from registrar interviews.

Category 1: Training or education

- Helpful = problem-based approach (teaching based on approaches to problems which are not limited to textbooks).
- Less helpful = emphasis on managing disease (teaching focused on current policies for disease management).

In the early days of their work, registrars wanted some factual teaching to help them find their feet in general practice:

'I think to begin with it was useful looking at disease management, sort of mild things you don't come across in hospital.'

But after a very short while the majority of trainees found that disease management teaching began to miss the spot:

'We did hypertension and asthma and all those things but it was the general problem-solving that I found more helpful.'

Ways that GPs preferred their teaching:

- *Concentrating* on problem-solving approaches, not facts that can be found in textbooks.
- *Emphasising* 'that you don't need to know *everything* about everything'.
- *Demonstrating* methodical approaches that translate across different problem areas.
- *Exploring* widely in learning – beyond the confines of the surgery.
- *Modelling* how to think beyond the obvious and to think laterally.
- *Teaching* about the process of keeping up to date and choosing what is relevant.

'To be trained is to have arrived – to be educated is to continue to travel' (Calman, 1994). Marinker (1992) expanded on the qualities delineated in this category:

'Training simply prepares the learner to perform tasks already identified and described, by methods which have gained general approval. Training teaches us to solve puzzles not to solve problems. Education teaches us to solve problems, the nature of which may not be known at the time when the education is taking place, and the solutions to which cannot be seen or even imagined by the teachers.' (Marinker, 1992, pp. 75–80)

Registrars were pressed for examples of tutorials where the approach turned out to be of lasting value:

'There was actually, it was one about rheumatoid arthritis and what was interesting was not necessarily the topic but for some reason it broke down the anxieties I had about having to help patients live with their chronic disorders.'

Another example:

'I had a real thing about contraception in terms of feeling I knew absolutely nothing at all and I hadn't the first idea about how to go about counselling someone about contraception. My trainer took me very methodically through a kind of how-to consult on contraception. And I remember feeling "Thank God I've got something in terms of a framework to work on".'

There was a lot of osmotic learning (Claxton, 1997) in the sessions that were of lasting value:

'And so our debates would sort of run into these questions and without knowing it you gained all that experience of thinking through problems.'

Exercise: Think of the last tutorial you took part in (either as tutor or tutee). How would you rate it on this spectrum? Was there any discussion about approaches which could be of lasting value long after current disease-management policies have been superseded?

Category 2: Style spectrum

- Helpful = wide variety of styles (learner exposed to different consulting styles and role-models in tutorials).
- Less helpful = narrow range of styles (teaching dominated by personal style and behaviour of trainer).

The former registrars were unanimous in valuing the wider variety of styles. Of lasting help were the following.

- Learning that there is not a single 'right way' of doctoring; a misconception sometimes arising from previous didactic hospital teaching.
- Joint consulting sessions with all the doctors in the practice throughout the year, not just 'sitting in' at the beginning.
- A culture valuing difference in the practice.
- Working alongside non-doctors, as well as doctors consulting, helps to define the contribution of the doctor.

One registrar put his finger on the value of a broad style spectrum:

'The fact that you can approach a problem in different ways with your own style and still come out with the same answer.'

'I can still be me and approach it in my way but actually still give the patient what they need.'

'I think general practice is such a melting pot, there's so many different approaches – they're all valid and right but it just helps to think more broadly if you've been taught more broadly.'

HPE point

If close observation of a broad range of styles is valuable to young doctors, and if they benefit from 'trying on hats to see if they fit', how can they broaden their experience in HPE? Are there opportunities for GPs to gain work experience in other settings?

> **Example 1**
>
> Sally, who trained in a rural practice, close to where she is now working, has little experience of working with ethnic minorities. She has only a few Asian families on her list, but feels she is not giving them the best service. A day's attachment to an inner-city practice with an Asian link-worker gave her new ideas for her own practice.
>
> **Example 2**
>
> Kumar identified a lack of confidence consulting with patients with enduring mental illness. He had never done a psychiatry job, and came across little serious mental illness in his training practice, but now finds himself working in a practice with several 'care-in-the-community' patients. Half a day spent sitting in with each of consultant psychiatrist, a CPN and a section-12 approved GP has done a lot to extend his repertoire of consulting behaviours with these patients and to improve his confidence.

Category 3: Space for reflection

- Helpful = encouraging reflective practitioner (safe environment to learn from mistakes).
- Less helpful = protocol-driven behaviour (black and white approach adopted where learner is expected to adhere to guidelines and elements of blame culture likely).

Challenge is very different from blame and challenge is essential to nurturing reflection, and welcomed by learners.

Teaching behaviours that promoted reflective thinking:

- trainers modelling self-challenge
- questioning accepted doctrines
- creating time and space for reflection in the working day
- promoting a no-blame culture through significant event analysis
- lateral thinking approaches
- effective use of silence in tutorials
- trainers not coming up with answers to registrars' dilemmas, but eliciting internal resources from the learner, by judicious Socratic questioning
- avoiding protocols wherever possible!

There is a rather uncomfortable paradox here about protocol-driven behaviour. It is a generally accepted aspect of 'good practice' that doctors conform to accepted protocols and guidelines in their behaviour (Wensing *et al.*, 1998) and yet our research suggests the most helpful behaviour in training practices is encouragement for learners to reflect rather than immediate reference to protocols and guidelines. Later, it may be helpful to refer to guidelines but they can have a stifling effect on reflection if they are the automatic response to questions brought up by learners.

In Accident and Emergency, the consultant, who has responsibility for the actions of many junior doctors, has often written protocols to ensure that there is a standard safe therapeutic action for a given clinical situation. In the more autonomous situation of general practice, different supervisory behaviour is required of trainers if learners are to become truly patient-centred.

Encouraging and guiding reflection is central to both the vocational training scheme agenda and the HPE learning that follows. Unless young doctors have reflective learning modelled and developed at this stage, it is unlikely that they will acquire the skills needed for continuing life-long learning.

Recent work on the stage theory of 'how doctors learn' has suggested that there is a preliminary phase of scanning:

> 'The doctor is aware that problems are "out there". The doctor is alert for problems which he might need to solve and, when potential problems are encountered, he moves on to the next stage.'

(Slotnick, 1999)

Good vocational training should ensure GP registrars are at Slotnick's 'Learning Stage 0' and ready to progress with life-long learning. Herein lies the importance of modelling personal development in the training practice, which is the basis of our next category (Category 4).

Category 4: Modelling personal development and teams

- Helpful = personal development and team management skills taught (guided learning of skills such as time management, assertiveness, boundary-setting).
- Less helpful = no emphasis on team behaviours (little attempt is made to help learner understand the importance of team-working and the areas of personal development that are involved).

This category is broad, almost to the point of being diffuse, but after much debate it was decided that the benefits of integration into a single category outweighed the risk of not separating potentially distinct entities. Thus, it may be argued that where GPs are learning advanced skills of time management, this affects their team behaviours and, indeed, it is not a good idea to consider time management in isolation.

As a simple example, the way one doctor chooses to deal with telephone consultations affects both the other partners and the reception staff, as well as the patients. In learning to adapt their behaviours to take account of the needs of others, and at the same time to be aware of the importance of self preservation, doctors are on a journey of personal development.

Helpful teaching behaviours on surviving and thriving in teams:

- Personal development and team management skills are taught explicitly.
- Guided learning of skills such as time management, assertiveness, boundary-setting.
- Special attention on how, when and why to say 'no'!
- Not merely allowing registrars to attend contentious or confidential meetings, but making explicit the underlying issues and attitudes.
- Developing a culture of openness throughout the practice, so that the behaviour of others can be constructively and reciprocally critiqued.

- Explicit discussion of home/work life-balance issues.
- Discussing values.
- Maintaining genuine enthusiasm for the job.

As indicated previously, it is crucial that trainers are aware of the power of their personal modelling. It is not necessary for trainers to be paragons of excellence to model effectively; what is needed is for them to be aware of the effects of their attitudes and behaviours on registrars, and to demonstrate the ways in which they are addressing their own personal and professional development within the practice context.

Category 5: Learning cycles

- Helpful = learning cycles completed (a culture exists in the practice where reflection, audit, assessment all promote change and re-evaluation).
- Less helpful = haphazard change (culture is reactive to external pressures, and little evidence of information about the practice inspiring meaningful change).

Interviews with former registrars endorsed the lasting value that is placed on an evidence-based culture where audit and assessment help to complete learning cycles. Many commented on the difficulty of completing audit cycles within a year, a problem that has been subsequently addressed in changing summative assessment from the five-point audit to the eight-point audit, allowing the effect of change to be assessed.

Helpful educational practice:

- Gives real meaning and value to audit, for example reference by the practice to changes made in response to previous registrars' audit projects.
- Promotes explicit change management along sound theoretical lines.
- Encourages pro-activity rather than reactivity.

The importance of cycles in learning and audit has been a recurrent theme in the literature since the time of Kolb (Kolb and Fry, 1975), so it is interesting that GP learners emphasise the importance of completing cycles. Slotnick (1999) puts it somewhat differently in his work on 'how doctors learn'. He concentrates on a stage theory (breaking each stage down to the *goals*, the *discrepancy* resolved during the stage, the way *learning resources* are used, the *reflection* during the stage and the *criteria* for successful completion).

HPE point

Not every registrar will have had positive experience of audit in their vocational training, yet all should have acquired the skills to conduct a successful audit, in order to pass summative assessment. Now is perhaps the time to put these skills to good use and to embed the practice of meaningful audit into life-long practice. Using protected HPE time to look intelligently at an aspect of practice, and to follow this up with practical change management, will not only benefit HPE learners, but will also bring tangible rewards to the practice that has supported the protected time for HPE learning.

Category 6: Family practice in context

- Helpful = contextualised learning (trainer introduces the broader dimensions of family and health expectations).
- Less helpful = emphasis on presenting problem (focus remains on sorting and shifting).

Registrars have selected family practice often on account of an interest in the broader family and social dimensions of medicine. It is perceived as vital that trainers teach about the context of family medicine:

'What I certainly learnt from my training practice was that looking at the individual as they came in as a member of the family and knowing more about their social context helped in a lot of the diagnostic processes.'

Helpful behaviours include:

- Importing knowledge of the wider family into problem case analysis.
- Encouraging reception and nursing staff to talk to registrars about patients and their backgrounds.
- Imaginative multi-cultural awareness teaching.
- Encouraging registrars to think about the occupational and school implications of patients' illnesses.

'It took a year for me to really work out that I did like patients and after all want to chat to them all day. And see the patient as the important thing rather than the disease or diagnostics or anything else,' said one former registrar, in what, perhaps, is a rather oversimplified view. But the point remains that if we want to retain doctors in general practice, we have to develop a fascination with what 'makes patients tick', for therein lies much of our professional enjoyment.

HPE point

New principals and salaried doctors in long-term posts may be struggling as they take on responsibility for a patient list for the first time. Part of the burden could be the newness of 'whole-family' medicine, whereby family members bring their troubles to the GP. Many doctors emerge from vocational training never having had husbands/wives, partners/lovers, adolescent sons/fathers, middle-aged daughters/elderly mothers consecutively bring their respective problems into the consulting room. Who to believe? How much to intervene? What are the doctor's responsibilities?

But family medicine is not only a problem – it can be a solution. This may be an example of where HPE learners could use an established course, such as the year-long weekly day-release course in family systems thinking at the Tavistock Clinic, to direct their life-long learning and their clinical practice along new lines.

Category 7: Control and direction

- Learner-centred approach (trainer listens to trainee and positively seeks out their educational needs, adapting the training accordingly).
- Trainer-centred approach (trainer adopts rigid structure with fixed views on the educational diet to feed trainees).

There are some distinctions to be drawn here between learner-centred education and learner-directed education. Good education can be learner-centred whoever directs it, but learners valued an increasing role in directing their education as the year progressed, whatever their starting point on the scale of dependence to independence as a learner.

Helping learners to become self-directing: reflecting back on the process, former registrars found it helpful when trainers:

- Ensured teaching is relevant and interesting.
- Responded to needs rather than just to wants.
- Maintained a sense of direction and purpose in teaching.
- Demonstrated flexibility in curriculum planning.
- Agreed to disagree when appropriate.
- Matched support and challenge.
- Most importantly, ensured learners felt valued at all times.

By the time that learners embark on an HPE programme, it is assumed that they are self-directed in their learning. What, then, are the roles for HPE tutors? We shall return to this later in Chapter 6, but in the meantime it may be appropriate to reflect on what former vocational training scheme registrars have taught us about the skills of educational supervision and mentoring.

Category 8: Feedback

- Sensitive feedback (both positive and negative feedback delivered where appropriate, stimulating confidence in the learner, and encouraging change).

- Inappropriate criticism (feedback either inadequate or mis-placed or poorly delivered, often not timely or specific enough to be useful to learner).

This category was almost omitted on the grounds that it is rather stating the obvious. But to have left out feedback would have meant being unfaithful to the principle of grounded theory, namely to seek out and report what the research data was saying. Loud and clear, time and again, interviewees emphasised the importance of good feedback.

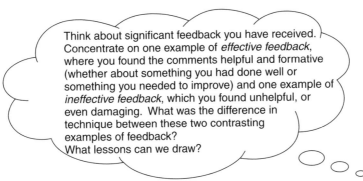

Think about significant feedback you have received. Concentrate on one example of *effective feedback*, where you found the comments helpful and formative (whether about something you had done well or something you needed to improve) and one example of *ineffective feedback*, which you found unhelpful, or even damaging. What was the difference in technique between these two contrasting examples of feedback? What lessons can we draw?

There was nothing new in what the interviewees had to say about effective feedback. They wanted it frequently and to be:

- timely
- specific
- constructive.

Learners who felt they had an honest triangulated picture of their performance appeared to be more comfortable in their learning.

Pulling the threads together

So what are the important educational features of vocational training? Educationalists have begun to tease out some relevant factors. Bligh (1992) suggested three principal factors influenced GP trainees' readiness to learn.

1   Enjoyment and enthusiasm for learning.
2   A positive self-concept as a learner.
3   A reproducing orientation to learning.

The responses in the interviews we conducted were mostly positive for these factors, and suggest that those doctors interviewed were potentially receptive learners.

A Delphi study (Munro *et al.*, 1998) carried out in South Thames with GP trainers, registrars and non-training principals looked for key attributes of GP trainers and revealed four factors.

1   Interpersonal relationships.
2   Professional development.
3   Personality.
4   Teaching quality.

It would seem that Category 1 (training or education) alongside Category 4 (modelling personal development and teamworking) are of prime importance in respect of these attributes, but it is likely that Category 7 (flexibility) and Category 8 (feedback) are also highly relevant.

Consider, lastly, some quotes from our interviews that exemplify the qualities which Munro *et al.* (1998) are describing:

'After eight years of doing hospital jobs then I had one year in practice and my whole approach to people was completely changed by my year in practice. And it was quite incredible really, I feel it certainly changed my whole approach to consultation and everything.'

'What training needs to do for you is to give you an idea what the job's going to be like; to deal with situations which you wouldn't normally deal with – maybe the wider family or the added-on baggage; make sure you're looking at what you are doing and why you are doing it.'

'In a roundabout way, as I sit in my office now, I reflect back on the training year and I think they did do their best to prepare me for most things that I've actually encountered – credit where it's due really.'

If vocational training has been successful, this is the starting point for HPE.

References

Bligh JG (1992) Independent learning among general practice trainees: an initial survey. *Medical Education* **26**, 497–502.

Calman K (1994) The profession of medicine. *British Medical Journal* **309**, 1140–1143.

Claxton G (1997) *Hare Brain, Tortoise Mind*. Fourth Estate, London.

Crawley HS and Levin JB (1990) Training for general practice: result of a survey into the general practitioner trainee scheme. *British Medical Journal* **300**, 911–915.

Gallen D and Buckle G (2001) *Personal and Practice Development Plans in Primary Care*. Butterworth Heinemann, Oxford.

Grow G (1991) Teaching learners to be self-directed. *Adult Education Quarterly* **41**, 125–149.

Hindmarsh JH, Coster GD *et al*. (1998) Are vocationally trained general practitioners better GPs? A review of research designs and outcomes. *Medical Education* **32**, 244–254.

Johnson N, Hasler J *et al*. (1997) The role of a practice manager in training practice assessment visits. *Education for General Practice* **8**, 128–134.

Joint Committee on General Practice Training (JCGPT) (2001) *Recommendations on the Selection of General Practice Trainers*. Joint Committee on General Practice Training, London.

Kolb D and Fry R (1975) Towards an applied theory of experiential learning. In: C Cooper, *Theories of Group Processes*. Wiley, London, 33–54.

Marinker M (1992) Assessment of postgraduate medical education – future directions. In: M Lawrence and P Pritchard (eds) *General Practitioner*

Education, UK and Nordic Perspectives. Springer Verlag, London, 75–80.

Munro N, Hornung R *et al.* (1998) What are the key attributes of a good general practice trainer? *Education for General Practice* **9**, 263–270.

Peile E, Easton G *et al.* (2001) The year in a training practice: what has lasting value? *Medical Teacher* **23**, 205–211.

Rethans J-J and Saebu L (1977) Do general practitioners act consistently in real practice when they meet the same patient twice? Examination of intradoctor variation using standardised (simulated) patients. *British Medical Journal* **314**, 1170.

Schofield T and Hasler J (1984a) Approval of trainers and training practices in the Oxford region: assessment. *British Medical Journal* **288**, 612–614.

Schofield T and Hasler J (1984b) Approval of trainers and training practices in the Oxford region: evaluation. *British Medical Journal* **288**, 618–619.

Schofield T and Hasler J (1984c) Approval of trainers and training practices in the Oxford region: criteria. *British Medical Journal* **288**, 538–540.

Slotnick H (1999) *How Doctors Learn.* Annual Meeting, Sussex, UK.

Wensing M, van der Weijden T *et al.* (1998) Implementing guidelines and interventions in general practice: which interventions are effective? *British Journal of General Practice* **48**, 991–997.

3

Vocational training: the bits that vocational training does not reach (identifying the gaps)

Introduction

This chapter considers the gaps in the vocational training scheme as they have been identified by 39 newly qualified GPs. It also compares the ideas of 33 trainers and course organisers. Lastly, it examines how, if at all, these educational needs could influence the vocational training scheme curriculum. The work was carried out in the Oxford Deanery during 2001–2002, and although it was a local study covering four counties, the findings are reflected nationally.

Orme-Smith (1998) describes the aim of GP vocational training as being to equip those entering general practice with the skills, knowledge and understanding to practise independently. An aim which is echoed by deaneries across the country. However, Styles (1990) suggests that the vocational training does not prepare newly qualified GPs for all the experiences they may face in the transition from registrar to principal. This theme is frequently reiterated throughout the literature on the subject:

'The first few years as a principal can be full of uncertainty, change and insecurity.' (Gallen *et al.*, 1994)

'VTS no longer adequate to meet the needs of an intending GP.'

(Hibble, 1996)

'There is a feeling of being lost at the end of training and experiencing a void.'

(Bonsor *et al.*, 1998)

'There is a transition period after becoming a new principal and before becoming a competent independent GP.'

(Smith *et al.*, 2000)

In 1994 the RCGP expressed its view that vocational training should help GPs to deal with the many changes they will encounter. In preparing new GPs for future responsibilities vocational training should enable them not only to manage change but, when needed, to initiate change. Much has also been written about the length of vocational training and where it should take place. As far back as 1968 the Royal Commission on Medical Education (RCME, 1968) expressed a need for longer training for general practice vocational training schemes. The World Health Organization (1995) expressed the view that most GP vocational training should be primary care-oriented and based in general practice. Although some schemes have now extended to 18 months in general practice many still continue with the traditional 12 months. It appears that little has changed in the last 30 years.

What, then, causes concern? What should GP registrars learn on the vocational training scheme and clearly fail to do so? Several studies have been conducted to identify why GP registrars feel that they end their vocational training with 'unfinished business'.

Key (1985), Berrington *et al.* (1996), Bonsor *et al.* (1998) and Dixon and van Zwanenberg (2001) all cite the following predominant gaps in vocational training:

- practice management
- multiprofessional working/teamwork

- medical audit
- use of computers
- NHS evolution and priorities.

The same themes have been recurrent over many years. They do not reflect areas of clinical need but focus on areas of organisation and management. Gallen and Buckle (1997) argue that whilst vocational training recognises the need to develop these skills it often struggles to win over the audience. This is sometimes due to the lack of a clearly defined management curriculum. It is also because it is often not until GPs have become principals that the impact and importance of the topics descends upon them.

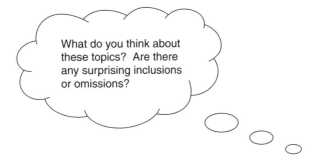

What do you think about these topics? Are there any surprising inclusions or omissions?

Assessing needs to identify gaps

The following study reflects work undertaken in the Oxford Deanery between October 2001 and July 2002. The aim of the work was to consider how HPE could be used effectively by the first cohort of learners able to access this initiative. It would be all too easy to assume that the needs of newly qualified GPs at the beginning of the twenty-first century were an exact reflection of what was found in the literature. It would then have been equally easy to organise a series of seminars or courses and hope there had been sufficient publicity and that our HPE learners took advantage of the opportunities offered. However, to assume that newly qualified GPs are aware of the HPE initiative and have consciously identified their learning needs is an assumption too far. It is important for individuals to acknowledge their learning needs and to have 'ownership' of the developing HPE programme. In order to do this they need to be involved in the needs assessment process.

Newly qualified GPs were asked to answer 18 open questions covering the areas listed below. They were also invited to attend a focus group to enable them to elaborate on their written statements. Course organisers and trainers were sent a similar questionnaire.

- Practice management and finance.
- Teamwork.
- Information technology and audit.
- Project management and research and development.
- Organisations, national service frameworks and health improvement programmes.
- Clinical topics.

We recognise that similar studies have been and will be carried out across different deaneries and suspect that their findings will not be dissimilar to ours. However, the purpose of this chapter is to consider the learning needs of newly qualified GPs rather than to compare the different approaches taken by each deanery.

Practice management and finance

Q1   During your training period what areas of practice management did you learn about?

Q2   Give examples of practice finance and budgeting in which you feel confident.

Q3   In what areas of practice management does your knowledge need to be developed further?

Q4   What further area of finance would you like covered?

Q5   Thinking about non-clinical skills needed by a GP, are there any areas in which you would like further training or development?

Q6   Are there any areas of your personal development that you feel you need more help with in order to manage your professional responsibilities effectively?

Response from potential HPE learners

The level of learning about practice management varies from quite considerable training to little or none at all. Most learners have received tutorials about:

- Basic areas of practice finance, such as items of service claims and other areas covered by the statement of fees and allowance.
- The role of the practice manager.
- The role of the GP as an employer, including staff recruitment and personnel matters.
- Health and safety.

However, most newly qualified GPs say they are not confident in areas of practice management and frequently highlight knowledge of practice finance as a major area for concern. Specific areas of finance are: budgetary control with regard to income and expenditure; partnership finances; and new government initiatives. Staff management, recruitment and development, and dealing with poor performance are also highlighted as learning needs in this area. Other non-clinical skills considered to be very desirable are leadership, negotiating, assertiveness, management of change and time management.

Response from the focus group

The focus group emphasised the need to understand the organisational aspects of practice and partnership in order to make the transition from registrar to partner. Non-principals also feel these to be important areas for further development in order for them to contribute to the practices in which they worked.

Lecture format is not considered a useful way to address this learning need. Reading about the subject is also not enough. The suggested format is the development of action learning sets and the encouragement of problem-based learning. A useful resource for a learning set might be a principal with two to three years' experience, a knowledgeable practice manager, and an accountant and a solicitor – both with experience in dealing with practice finance and partnership issues.

Response from course organisers and trainers

Trainers and course organisers vary in what they feel has been covered adequately. However, most considered that finance had been covered, though some felt it was an area which needed further development after vocational training.

Comments from course organisers and trainers

Much of what is taught or learnt under this heading appears to depend on the particular interest of the registrar:

'You can take a horse to water but you can't make it drink'

or the particular circumstances of the training practice:

'There was a change of practice manager'

'No one in the practice has any expertise in PMS'

or even whether it was considered appropriate to vocational training:

'Most of these topics have little application and will be forgotten until the registrars are partners.'

Teamwork

Q7 Teamwork is clearly important. What training has helped you develop your teamwork?

Q8 In what way could you further develop your teamwork skills?

Q9 What help do you need in developing your skills to be effective in different roles at meetings?

Response from potential HPE learners

All respondents acknowledge the importance of teamwork and feel they have been exposed to both positive and negative experiences in this area. They do, however, require further understanding of how teams work, how to develop teams and how to deal with dysfunctional teams. They also recognised the importance of developing skills for chairing meetings and improving their understanding of group dynamics. Learning how to give constructive feedback and how to deal with conflict during meetings is also highlighted as a learning need.

Response from the focus group

It was felt that whilst some skills, such as chairing meetings, could be learnt from attending a course a great deal may be learnt by observation so long as there is some knowledge of the theory behind teamwork and group dynamics.

Response from course organisers and trainers

Course organisers and trainers feel that the importance of teamwork is well covered through practical demonstrations and experience within the training practice. However, they accept that registrars could benefit from learning more about the theory of teamwork. This would enable them to understand why some teams were dysfunctional and give them team building skills to use in their own practice. They suggest that registrars have an active role in practice meetings, which enables them to learn through observing the behaviours of others so long as there is formal reflection.

Information technology and audit

Q10   In what areas of information technology (IT) are you less confident?
Q11   How could your IT skills be developed?
Q12   How can your audit skills be developed to enable you to undertake effective audit?

Response from potential HPE learners

Most respondents defined IT as understanding both commercial and clinical software. Some also defined IT as having an understanding about hardware. Some individuals have fairly advanced computer skills and want to improve their ability to design web pages. Others, however, feel they have very limited skills and that they have much to learn about all aspects of IT. The majority of HPE learners feel their IT skills are basic but adequate, though many suggest areas in which they would like to improve. These areas include internet searches, the use of specific software, such as PowerPoint, Excel and Access, and a better understanding of computer hardware.

The limited understanding of the clinical software system is often given as an inhibiting factor to undertaking audit within the practice. Improving skills in the development of templates and searches might give some newly qualified GPs more confidence in undertaking clinical or organisational audits. However, computer skills are not the only limiting factor. Time is perceived as a major issue, as protected time is rarely set aside for the purpose of audit.

Response from the focus group

The comments made by the focus group particularly emphasise the problems concerning clinical coding, the frustration of searching the clinical database and the frequent resistance to audit within the practice as a whole. They suggest that computer skills must be learnt in a 'hands-on' fashion. One-to-one teaching is preferable, although computer 'labs' where each student has their own machine may also be an option. They feel that clinical systems require 'on the job' learning. This may require a trainer from the computer company or someone from the practice (or another practice) with the necessary knowledge and teaching skills. Sharing 'best practice' across a primary care trust could also be a useful way to maximise the use of the clinical system.

Promoting the importance of audit is considered to be almost as important as developing the skills to undertake audit and that this might be a role for the primary care trust. The use of audit facilitators employed by the primary care trusts as an expert resource is also a possible way of developing skills. However, it was recognised that such experts should be developmental and supportive in order for others to learn, rather than them undertake an audit on their behalf.

Response from course organisers and trainers

Some course organisers and trainers feel that it is now reasonable to expect registrars to have a sound basic understanding of computers before they join the vocational training scheme. Others suggest that obtaining the European computer driving licence (ECDL) is a useful tool with which to develop computer skills. Developing skills for the clinical system appears to be on a 'need to know' basis unless registrars have a particular interest in this area. Course organisers and trainers consider audit to be well covered during vocational training, with the requirement of audit for summative assessment providing a focal point. Some trainers feel that registrars are encouraged to consider the practical implementation of audit but for others the importance of the audit cycle was not stressed sufficiently.

Comments from course organisers and trainers

'They must think about the process of care and not just audit as an exercise.'

'They need to understand the relationship between audit and mananging change.'

'It is important to know the difference between an audit and a survey.'

Many trainers and course organisers acknowledge the problems with accessing data and the detrimental effect this often has on the effectiveness of the audit.

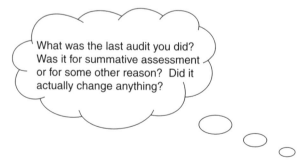

What was the last audit you did? Was it for summative assessment or for some other reason? Did it actually change anything?

Project management and research and development

Q13   Do you have experience in research and development (R&D); if so please describe what you have done.
Q14   What is your understanding of project management?
Q15   Do you need to develop your skills in project management?

Response from potential HPE learners

Few HPE learners have any experience in research and development and most are not interested in pursuing it. It was not considered to be an important area for development unless it was of particular interest to the individual. Project management was considered by everyone to be an important area for development. Half of our potential HPE learners felt they have some skills but need further development, whereas the other half said they had no project management skills at all.

Response from the focus group

Those who wished to develop skills in R&D did so because they felt it would be a useful dimension to their career as a GP. It was recognised that such skills would probably be developed by undertaking research under appropriate supervision. Project management is considered to be an important area for development. It would help to improve confidence in undertaking project work within a practice. Some felt that undertaking a successful project would help to 'establish' themselves within the practice. A workshop format is thought to be an appropriate way of addressing this need.

Response from course organisers and trainers

It was felt that R&D skills would only be developed if registrars had a real interest in the area. It was also felt that there was insufficient time during the normal vocational training period to cover R&D.

Comments from course organisers and trainers

'R&D skills are not really important. I feel it is easier for a busy GP to review articles where the appraisal has been done by an expert.'

'They are desirable but not essential to be regarded as minimally competent.'

'They [registrars] only need to know enough to do a basic audit.'

'Critical appraisal skills are important for evaluation.'

Many felt that registrars are actively involved in project management but that there is little specific teaching of the skills involved. Where skills are taught it tends to be as part of the centralised vocational training sessions rather than by the trainer or member of the training practice.

Organisations, NSFs and HImPs

Q16   What work have you done concerning a national service framework (NSF) or health improvement programme (HImP)?

Q17   Do you feel you have sufficient understanding of the following to enable you to contribute to practice development:
      – primary care organisations

- personal medical services (PMS) and general medical
  services (GMS)
- intermediate care
- GP with special interest (GPwSI)
- clinical governance?

Response from potential HPE learners

Everyone was aware of national service frameworks but few
had any direct experience of either working with the guidelines
or being involved in their implementation within their training
practice. However, less than half had sufficient understanding
of primary care organisations, GPs with special interests and
intermediate care to feel they could make an informed decision
or useful contribution to a practice discussion on the subjects.
None of the respondents had knowledge of health improvement
programme priorities. Most had a reasonable understanding of
what clinical governance was about, although few had first-
hand experience of being involved with developing the practice
policies. The degree of experience appears to be related to
the degree in which the training practice is involved with the
'initiatives', for example having a partner who is the clinical
governance lead for a primary care organisation.

Response from the focus group

The group again stressed that whilst it recognised the importance
of many of these issues it felt 'disconnected' from the process
and overwhelmed by the agendas. This was particularly true of
national service frameworks, health improvement programmes
and clinical governance. The group was concerned with having
insufficient understanding to either implement or support implementation within the practice.

The organisational issues – primary care organisations, inter-mediate care and PMS/GMS – are considered to be important but less urgent as they are thought to be part of the evolution of the health service. However, we need to develop a mechanism for bringing HPE learners up to date with these issues and also to develop transferable skills, which may be applied to the imple-mentation of other initiatives.

Response from course organisers and trainers

It was generally agreed that there was little or no development of registrars' knowledge in these areas during the vocational training period. Where it does occur it again reflects a training practice where another team member was actively involved in the initiative.

Comments from course organisers and trainers

'Involvement with a partner who is at the heart of these initiatives.'

'Attending PCG meetings [with involved partner] as an observer.'

Clinical topics

Q18   What areas of clinical skill and knowledge would you like to develop further?

Response from potential HPE learners

Between them the respondents listed 20 different clinical areas in which they would like to improve their skills; some listed more than one area, dermatology being listed 10 times and paediatrics and minor operations each listed six times.

Response from the focus group

The group acknowledged the diversity of the clinical areas requiring further development and recognised that these would be better addressed on a personal basis. Addressing these needs could be done in a number of ways, including:

- attendance at out-patients clinics
- clinical assistant posts
- journal clubs
- e-learning
- conferences/workshops/seminars.

It was agreed that the HPE tutors would act as 'sign posts' for individuals with clinical needs and would not organise specific training sessions on clinical topics.

Response from course organisers and trainers

No specific clinical skills were highlighted. It was felt that all clinical areas could be further developed but that this would happen with time.

Views from course organisers and trainers

Course organisers and trainers felt there was a need for newly qualified GPs to have 'formal' support mechanisms in the early post-qualification period. This is not so much to develop in specific areas, but to enable them to do more than 'survive'. Areas for concern included handling uncertainty; balancing home, work and leisure; making time for own educational needs; coping with stress and avoiding burn-out. These views were also similar to those of the HPE learners, who emphasised the importance of being able to access support both from their peer group and if possible a mentor.

It was generally felt that the vocational training scheme year was already very full and that not all topics could be covered in depth.

'Most topics need introduction but equally most will be refined with experience.'

'Practice management only makes sense if you have a practice to manage.'

'I try to ensure that registrars have a taster of everything, so they can decide what they want to develop further after their training.'

'Have you lot never heard of life-long learning?'

Overall, the group felt that their specific objectives for the vocational training period were:

'To turn out a clinically competent doctor.'

'To prepare them for a "never ending journey".'

'To encourage enthusiasm for life-long learning.'

'To be an effective and caring independent practitioner.'

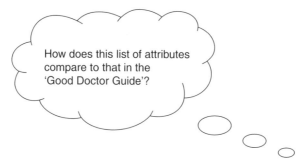

How does this list of attributes compare to that in the 'Good Doctor Guide'?

Course organisers and trainers acknowledged that all the topics raised by the HPE learners were valid and that further development in these areas will be useful to new GPs.

Comparison of the views of learners and educators

There is little dissent between the gaps identified by HPE learners and those identified by the vocational training educators. There were, however, small differences as to the size of the gap in some of the topics.

Practice management and finance

This is perhaps the learning need which newly qualified GPs were most anxious to address. Course organisers and trainers also acknowledged this gap. However, many felt that they had tried to provide opportunities to address these topics during the vocational training scheme. They felt that very often registrars did not always engage in the topic as its relevance was not always apparent at the time of learning.

Teamwork

It was generally accepted that this was well covered during the vocational training period. However, there was also agreement that this was achieved implicitly through experiential learning. It was generally felt that explicit learning of underpinning theory would also be useful.

Audit and IT

This was the area where there was least agreement about how much has been and should be addressed during the registrar years. Course organisers and trainers felt that audit was well covered as a result of the need to complete summative assessment. Newly qualified GPs expressed opinions that although they had undertaken audit they had not necessarily developed the more technical IT skills which would make audit more effective. They were also concerned that undertaking a single audit did not always provide the skills needed in order to carry out an audit in a busy practice environment.

There was also a discrepancy in expectations of how much, by way of IT skills, registrars should be expected to possess when joining the vocational training scheme compared with what they should expect the vocational training scheme to teach them. Many HPE learners felt their IT skills to be badly lacking, whereas several course organisers and trainers felt that IT skills should be pursued outside the vocational training scheme.

Project management and R&D

The overriding opinion was that R&D was a useful but not essential skill. It was considered to be of greater importance for registrars who had a particular interest in the topic. It was not considered a core skill for newly qualified GPs.

Project management, however, was considered to be of more general importance. Much like audit, it was felt that projects had been undertaken during vocational training but without developing the underpinning and transferable skills that allow for effective project management within their own practice.

Organisations, NSFs and HImPs

There was agreement that whilst these are important areas of learning for new GPs they do not seem to form part of the vocational training scheme curriculum. The degree of exposure to these subjects was patchy and more by chance than design.

Clinical topics

Course organisers and trainers showed no surprise at the list of clinical topics. Both groups recognised that development in clinical areas will take time. They also acknowledged that development in the clinical areas will often be driven by the needs of a practice as well as the interests of individuals.

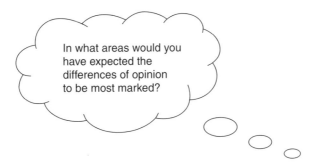

In what areas would you have expected the differences of opinion to be most marked?

What did we learn?

There was very little difference in the learning gaps identified by our potential HPE learners compared with previous studies and surveys on the subject. It appears that although some of the terminology may have changed, for example, 'fundholding' and 'FHSA' have now been replaced by PMS and primary care trust, the essence of what has been identified remains the same. However, the agenda has widened and now has to take account of government directives such as health improvement pro-grammes, national service frameworks and clinical governance – all of which affect practising GPs.

   The enormity and diversity of the agenda to be covered during the vocational training period is echoed throughout and, like previous studies, raises questions about the structure of vocational training as well as its content. Discussion about how much time should be spent doing what is not within the remit of this chapter. However, it is quite clear that HPE affords an opportunity to look at vocational training curriculum planning.

How should HPE influence the vocational training agenda?

It must be made clear at the outset that the need for HPE is not a criticism directed at those involved in GP vocational training. The development of HPE must be considered as a continuum of learning and an integral part of the learning continuum, that is, vocational training scheme–HPE–continuing professional development (life-long learning). The findings from this and other similar studies, along with the introduction of HPE, should enable GP educators to consider their curriculum development within vocational training schemes. This is not a case of how much more can we include in vocational training, but what is realistic and appropriate to the vocational training scheme and what is realistic and appropriate to HPE? It is essential that HPE is not regarded simply a mechanism for 'plugging' gaps, but develops its own curriculum as part of the educational continuum.

Summary

- GP registrars do feel a 'void' at the end of the vocational training scheme.

- Practice management and wider NHS organisational issues are identified as a greater learning need than clinical issues.

- Vocational training scheme course organisers and GP registrar trainers also acknowledge these gaps but not always to the same extent as the GP registrars.

- GP educators should work together to identify the role of vocational training and the role of HPE.

- HPE should be viewed as part of the continuum of life-long learning and not a mechanism to 'plug' gaps.

References

Berrington RM, Hibble AG and Sackin PA (1996) Higher professional education for general practice. *Education for General Practice* 7, 187–190.

Bonsor R, Gibbs T and Woodward R (1998) Vocational training and beyond – listening to voices from a void. *British Journal of General Practice* 48, 915–918.

Dixon H and van Zwanenberg T (2001) GP registrars' views on extending the general practice element of vocational training and higher professional education: a questionnaire study in the Northern deanery. *Education for General Practice* 12, 177–184.

Gallen D and Buckle G (1997) *Top Tips in Primary Care Management.* Blackwell Science, Oxford.

Gallen D, Coulson W and Buckle G (1994) *The First Steps in General Practice.* Blackwell Scientific Publications, Oxford.

Hibble A (1996) *Report of the First Cambridge Conference on Higher Professional Education for General Practice.* Cambridge, Anglia Region.

Key I (1985) Recruiting new principals in general practice. *British Medical Journal* 291, 451–455.

Orme-Smith A (1998) A new structure for GP vocational training. *Education for General Practice* 9, 173–178.

Royal Commission on Medical Education (1968) *Report cmnd 3569.* HMSO, London.

Smith L, Eve R and Crabtree R (2000) Higher professional education for general practitioners: key informant interviews and focus group findings. *British Journal of General Practice* 50, 293–299.

Styles W (1990) But now what? Some unsolved problems of training for general practice. *British Journal of General Practice* **40**, 270–276.

World Health Organization (1995) *A Charter for General Practice/Family Medicine in Europe*. WHO, Copenhagen.

4

Educational needs assessment

Introduction

HPE, like all adult learning, should reflect the needs of the learner. The aim of this chapter is to highlight the importance of educational needs assessment both for individuals and for the organisation. It also considers the effects of educational needs assessment on improving patient care. According to the *Good CPD Guide* (Grant *et al.*, 1999), educational needs assessment, or learning needs assessment, should be part of the process of all continuing professional development (CPD) and life-long learning. Equally, we would agree that not all learning will or must occur as a result of educational needs assessment (Grant, 2002). It is easy to assume that, as adult learners, doctors will be self-directed in their learning and automatically know how to identify their learning needs. However, this is not always the case and although much has been written about educational needs assessment the medical profession has not necessarily engaged in the process.

Definition

Defining an educational need, and therefore defining educational needs assessment, can be complex in itself. It is first useful to explore the definition of *need*, which may also be expressed as 'a want or a demand'. In 1972, Bradshaw produced his still frequently quoted taxonomy of need, in which he highlights four types of need:

- Normative need – defined by experts as a desirable standard.
- Felt need – defined by the individual who has the need.
- Comparative need – comparing one group with another.
- Expressed need – a felt need that is expressed by action.

For example, record-keeping:

- *Normative* – the General Medical Council (GMC) requires doctors to keep accurate clinical records.
- *Felt* – individual doctors feel they want to keep good records.
- *Comparative* – primary care organisations require all practices to keep records to a similar standard.
- *Expressed* – individual doctors keep additional records of patients' wishes.

The concept of 'need' can still be difficult to grasp owing to ambiguity in language. As a noun, *need* refers to the gap or discrepancy between the present state and the desired end state. *Need* is therefore neither the present nor the future state, but the gap between them. *Need*, as a verb, points to what is required or desired to fill the discrepancy, thus becoming the solution to the perceived problem.

For example, if we discuss our current staffing levels and then consider our desired staffing levels, the *need* (used as a noun) is the discrepancy between the two. However, we commonly discuss needing more doctors, more nurses and more hospitals, which when using *need* as a verb is a perceived solution to many problems. In this case the identified gap, that is, needing more doctors, nurses and hospitals, may then be taken up as the solution.

Therefore, a *need* may be defined as the discrepancy between current and desired states of being. An educational *need* for an HPE doctor may be that he or she has only limited IT skills but wishes to become more proficient in order to improve use of the computer during consultations.

For example: the *current* state is limited IT skills; the *desired* state is proficient use of the computer during consultations; the *need* is to learn how to use the computer.

The role of educational needs assessment is to determine such discrepancies, to examine their nature and cause, and to set priorities for future action. It may be defined as the *process* by which learners' educational needs are identified and diagnosed. Needs assessment should focus on the process of addressing gaps in skills and knowledge.

'Needs assessment' is a systematic set of procedures under-taken for the purpose of setting priorities and making decisions about programme or organisational improvement and allocation of resources. It can set the criteria for determining how best to allocate available resources. 'Learning needs assessment' will assist in planning and developing educational programmes and curricula. Needs assessment is also a process that HPE and other doctors have to undertake in order to provide healthcare for their practice populations. This will be discussed later in the chapter.

Phases of assessment

A needs assessment, educational or otherwise, is a systematic approach that progresses through a series of defined phases. Witkin (1995) outlines a useful three-phase model of needs assessment. These phases are pre-assessment, assessment and post-assessment.

Pre-assessment

The purpose of the pre-assessment phase is to investigate what is already known about the needs of the target group, to determine the focus and scope of the assessment and to gain commitment for all states of the assessment.

Assessment

The task of the assessment phase is to document status and compare this with the vision of what should be or is desirable. It should determine the magnitude of needs and their causes.

Post-assessment

In this phase, plans are made to use the information elicited in a practical way. What needs are most critical and why have they not been addressed previously? What are some of the possible solutions? This phase forms the bridge from analysis to action.

An example for HPE tutors might be:

- *Pre-assessment* – questionnaire and focus groups.
- *Assessment* – analysis of the above.
- *Post-assessment* – planning and prioritising to address gaps.

How do I know what I need to learn?

This is one of the questions most commonly asked by anyone trying to plan their educational and personal development. Answering the question is part of the needs assessment process. New GPs just completing their vocational training scheme may have no idea of the complexities of general practice. They will therefore not know what they need to know. Some of the gaps in clinical knowledge may become obvious as they see a variety of patients and conditions, and it is useful to keep a notebook recording these gaps. This will help to identify specific learning needs and also to identify any trends in learning needs, that is, several queries about skin conditions might highlight a need for improved understanding of dermatology.

Identifying non-clinical learning needs will follow a similar process. Initially, this will be prompted by a lack of understanding of a particular process, for example:

- How do I get paid?
- What goes to make up my monthly pay cheque?
- Why do we have such a high turnover of practice nurses?

There are many tools for educational needs assessment. These can be used by doctors or any other team members. They are also useful for looking at the needs of the practice as an organisation.

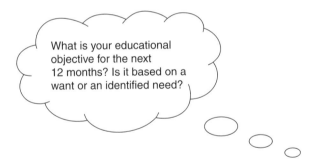

What is your educational objective for the next 12 months? Is it based on a want or an identified need?

Methods of educational needs assessment

Some of the methods used are very simple, whereas others are quite complex. Some methods are better-suited to individual use whilst others are useful in assessing group or organisational needs. This section will illustrate some of the many different tools. However, there is no definitive method and no one method ranks higher than another. Different methods will work better in different situations. Personal preference will be the key to highlighting the most effective methods for each individual.

Questionnaires

These can take the form of self-assessment or something that is collated by an external facilitator, either to be fed back to individuals or collectively to organisations. Questionnaires remain the most common method of needs assessment and are widely used in continuing professional education (Mann, 1998). There are, however, both advantages and disadvantages to this method.

Advantages:

- it is efficient in terms of materials and human resources, particularly if the target audience is large
- it can address a wide number of topics and can therefore assess the diverse educational needs of health professionals
- information may be returned in a standardised way
- it can be used in conjunction with other assessment tools, either to highlight areas which need further exploration or to focus on previously identified areas.

Disadvantages:

- a poorly designed questionnaire may be ignored by would-be respondents or, if completed, may not provide the intended information
- it cannot be assumed to be a valid and accurate representation of the population in question
- response rates are invariably low
- individuals vary in their ability to self-assess and therefore responses may not be accurate.

For example, a GP or practice nurse may complete a self-assessment questionnaire about the care of diabetic patients. If done solely, on an individual basis, it may highlight the learning needs of that individual. If all the health professionals in the practice complete the same questionnaire, the outcome might reveal an organisational need in care for diabetic patients in the practice.

Questionnaires clearly have a useful role to play in educational and organisational needs assessment. They can help to identify gaps between current and desired states. They can also provide information to influence personal and organisational planning.

Reflective diaries

These are similar to the notebook recording mentioned earlier in this chapter (*see* p. 64), but may be kept by any or all team members. It is therefore useful for identifying organisational as well as individual needs. A reflective diary is the means by which events over a set period of time are listed and analysed.

For example, for a doctor or nurse it could be their next 50 consultations; for a member of the administrative team it could be a reflection of the repeat prescribing process over five consecutive days. However, simply keeping a list is not enough. Individuals need to analyse this list to identify:

- trends or tendencies
- areas of potential error
- organisational deficiencies
- areas of strength.

They will then have to decide, possibly in discussion with others, how they will go about addressing these identified needs.

A reflective diary can be a very useful means of identifying learning needs – by highlighting what individuals did not know they needed to know.

Audit

Audit allows the practice or individuals to gain a clear picture of the current position, to decide what change is necessary, to implement the change and to review the action taken. Although audit is common practice for most doctors and their teams, it is less frequently recognised as a useful tool for educational needs assessment. Audit measures performance against specific pre-defined standards. Having identified the gap it can also give a good indication of the reason for the deficiency.

For example, comparing your disease register with those patients regularly prescribed the most appropriate or obvious medication can help to identify gaps in knowledge and in process. An audit undertaken to assess the prescribing of mebeverine for patients with a computer diagnosis of irritable bowel syndrome might show very low numbers. This could be due to a lack of up-to-date clinical knowledge on the subject. Alternatively, it could be due to the failure of one or more individuals to record information accurately. This audit may have highlighted both a clinical learning need and an IT learning need.

The audit itself will give figures and indicate performance in relation to standard. It is the questions that are then asked which give deeper insight into individual or organisational learning needs.

Interviews

An interview is described as a 'conversation with purpose'. For educational needs assessment that purpose is to gain in-depth insight into individuals' perspective and to acquire an in-depth appreciation of learners' practice environments and how that context shapes and influences performance. The interview process will form an integral part of the GP appraisal system, which if undertaken properly will also highlight learning and developmental needs.

Interviews may take place over the telephone, but the absence of visible body language often means that vital clues go undetected. For educational needs assessment a face-to-face interview is more desirable. The major advantage of the interview is that it is personal. Interviewers have an opportunity to elicit in-depth information that can lead to a greater understanding of individuals and their concerns. They can also expand on themes or clarify information gleaned from other sources (Bogdan and Bilken, 1992). The major disadvantage of interviews is the time that must be allowed for them and the process of getting interviewers and interviewees together at an appropriate time and setting. The skills of interviewers also play an important role in determining what information is elicited, that is, what learning needs have been identified and does the interviewee acknowledge them. It is essential to remember that the reason for undertaking an interview as part of educational needs analysis is to achieve in-depth understanding of the perceived and prescribed learning needs of individuals in their practice context. It is not appropriate to transfer conclusions to other environments as generalising is better achieved by other needs assessment methods.

Focus groups

This is a similar method to that of the interview. It is a method of group review that explicitly includes and uses group interaction to generate data. The use of focus groups for educational planning and learning needs assessment has been growing steadily over the last 30 years (Servier, 1989). The use of a focus group is a method for gathering a specific type of data and works well in providing educators with insights and clues as to how to develop programming or educational interventions. Specifically, focus groups provide a broader range of information than one-to-one interviews as members of the group draw 'strength' from one another and support the expression of ideas and opinions, some of which might be unpopular.

The disadvantage of focus groups is that they may not be representative of the target audience. They are often used, therefore, to complement other methods of needs assessment. Like interviews, focus groups can be very time-consuming and their success is equally dependent on skilled interviewers.

As the name implies, focus groups are a very useful method of gaining collective opinions and determining collective needs. They are very good for looking at organisational learning needs. Involving patients in focus groups will also provide a different perspective and, again, highlight gaps in knowledge of which the practice was unaware.

For example, a practice had a high number of patients with asthma but a low uptake in its asthma clinic, which was run by the only practice nurse qualified to do so. A focus group was formed, including patients who had asthma but who had not attended the clinic, all four members of the practice nurse team and a GP. It was facilitated by the practice manager. The findings were that patients did not attend because of the timing of the clinic, which was the only time the 'asthma nurse' could work. This highlighted an organisational need for the practice to consider. It also highlighted an educational need for at least one of the other practice nurses to undertake training in the care of patients with asthma.

In addition to use of a single focus group for a specific question, it is often useful to use multiple focus groups. This involves organising several groups, maybe from different disciplines or backgrounds. The use of multiple focus groups as a means of needs assessment can provide widely differing perspectives on the same subject.

Delphi technique

The name originates from the oracle at Delphi where the ancient Greeks were said to be able to forecast future events. In its current form, questionnaires are used in three successive iterations to aggregate the views of 'experts', allowing them to remain anonymous whilst preventing domination by particular individuals who may otherwise overly influence group discussions. Respondents are given feedback to each previous iteration of the study. This allows them to change their response completely, to maintain their previous position or to move towards consensus (Stritter *et al.*, 1994).

This method of needs assessment can be very useful when the issues are complex. However, it needs careful planning, not least to determine who the experts might be, and thus it is time-consuming. There is also a problem with respondents dropping out at any stage.

For example, the Delphi technique may be useful for looking at healthcare needs for a primary care organisation. The primary care organisation could start by asking members of each practice which services they feel they should provide for the primary care organisation and which additional services they could provide for the primary care organisation. This would enable the primary care organisation and the practices to reach consensus on what core services, and what additional services, are being provided by each practice. This, in turn, is likely to identify educational needs for the primary healthcare professionals in order to provide these services.

Nominal group technique

The nominal group technique is useful in gaining consensus from a wide range of people comparatively quickly. It is now considered to be superior to that of brainstorming (Stroebe and

Diehl, 1994). This method can also be a useful tool in needs assessment.

The technique involves asking a group of people each to commit their ideas on a given issue or topic to paper. This is done without discussion or conferring with others. The process is then as follows.

- Each participant is then asked to state what aspect of the problem or issue they personally consider to be the most important.
- These are then recorded on to a master sheet having clarified any ambiguous statements.
- Each statement is given a letter or number for easy identification.
- Each member of the group is now asked to rank the five issues that they personally consider to be the most important by scoring five points to the most important and one point to the least important.
- The information is collected from all participants and the result is tallied.
- The issue with the highest score is, by consensus, the most important issue for the whole team.

This method may be used within a practice or by the primary care organisation to consider organisational needs. In so doing, it may also highlight individuals' educational needs.

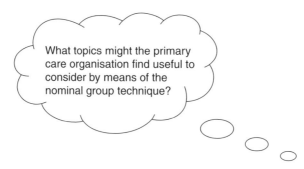

What topics might the primary care organisation find useful to consider by means of the nominal group technique?

Significant event analysis

Significant event analysis, sometimes referred to as 'critical incident review', is an essential part of risk assessment and risk management. It is also a useful method of educational needs assessment, both for individuals and for practices as organisations. A 'significant event' is any event that highlights a deficiency in individual doctors or in practice organisation and systems. However, we can also learn from a positive experience, such as some exceptional teamwork within the practice. It is the analysis of the significant event that provides the assessment process. It is important to track the event as far back as possible. This allows each step which led to the event itself to be examined. In doing so it may be seen where things started to go awry and at what stage, if any, the event could have been prevented. This may highlight a knowledge gap for individuals or it may highlight a collective knowledge and/or attitudinal gap for the practice as a whole.

For example, a patient with a very slightly suspect mole was seen by one of the GP principals and asked to book in for a minor ops clinic. A minor ops clinic is normally held at the practice each month. The patient was given a slip of paper, which read 'Next clinic please', to take to the reception desk. Unknown to the doctor who wrote the request the next two clinics had been cancelled owing to annual leave and a shortage of nurses in the treatment room. The receptionist did what was asked of her and booked the patient into the 'next' clinic which was in three months' time. By the time the patient attended the clinic the mole was more than a little suspicious. The GP decided to go ahead and excised the mole with a 3 mm margin. Sure enough, the mole turned out to be a malignant melanoma. The patient was referred to a consultant dermatologist, who pointed out, none too gently to the practice, that the departmental policy on suspicious moles was to take a 5 mm margin. In addition, he wanted to know why the patient had not been referred immediately to the dermatology department under the two-week cancer wait arrangements.

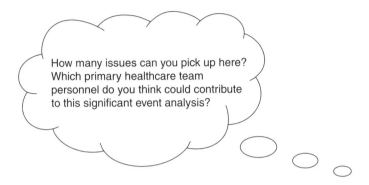

How many issues can you pick up here? Which primary healthcare team personnel do you think could contribute to this significant event analysis?

Patients' unmet needs and doctors' educational needs

Dr Richard Eve was the first to describe the use of patients' unmet needs (PUNs) and doctors' educational needs (DENs) (Eve, 2000) as a means of identifying educational needs during the consultation. Like some of the other methods we have mentioned these require keeping a record of the times when doctors feel that had they had more knowledge or understanding of a subject they could have improved their care of patients. By asking the question, 'How could I have done better?' they may identify an unmet need for patients. Identifying this need can then lead to the identification of doctors' learning needs.

360° feedback appraisals

Properly undertaken appraisal can be another useful and effective method of educational needs assessment. There are various methods of appraisal and although the interview stage is likely to be undertaken by another GP (DoH, 2001) appraisees can gather information about themselves, which will help to inform this process. A useful way of doing this is 360° feedback. This means that appraisees invite several people (11 is considered to be the optimum number) to give feedback on their competence, attitudes and professional relationships.

The concept of 360° is that individual feedback may come from anywhere in appraisees' circle of contacts, for example reception staff, nurses, health visitors, partners, hospital clinicians, etc. The feedback should be honest but constructive and may be anonymous. Undertaking a 360° feedback exercise may well highlight both strengths and weaknesses that appraisees had not considered previously. Highlighting strengths as well as being encouraging allows appraisees to prioritise their learning needs towards areas of weakness.

Personal development plans

Although educational needs assessment is an essential part of the personal development plan the review phase of the plan is itself a form of needs assessment. As they move from one year to the next health professionals will reconsider their learning needs in the light of the previous year's learning. The collective learning needs of all doctors and health professionals taken from their personal development plans, either across a practice or a primary care organisation, may also be valuable in informing the education programme for those groups.

For example, if several GPs have, through their personal development plans, identified a need to improve their knowledge on dermatology, the primary care organisation can maximise training resources by responding to the collective rather than individual learning need. The primary care organisation may work with educationalists and local dermatologists to organise training sessions specifically for GPs in that area.

The personal development plan is an excellent mechanism for capturing and pulling together all the identified learning needs from whatever methods of assessment have been chosen for use.

Educational needs assessment tools

- Questionnaires
- Reflective diaries
- Audit
- Interviews
- Focus groups
- Delphi technique
- Nominal group technique
- Significant event analysis
- PUNs and DENs
- 360° feedback
- Personal development plans.

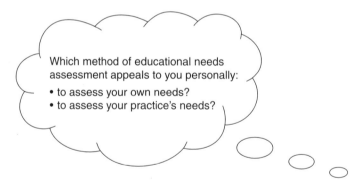

Which method of educational needs assessment appeals to you personally:

• to assess your own needs?
• to assess your practice's needs?

Understanding the health needs of the population

During this chapter we have, on several occasions, alluded to the use of needs assessment tools in assessing healthcare needs as well as educational needs. It is not unreasonable for the community as a whole, as well as individual patients, to expect the medical profession to provide a service that responds to its health needs. Therefore HPE and continuing professional development must acknowledge changing patterns of morbidity, changing political and economic climate and changing expectations from patients – all of which have a direct effect on patient care. This is clearly a wider remit than looking to plug gaps in a knowledge base.

Witkin (1995), who suggested the three phases of needs assessment, also suggests that needs assessment should be focused on the people in the system and illustrates this by thinking in terms of three levels of need.

- Level 1 (primary) – service-receivers.
- Level 2 (secondary) – service-providers and policy-makers.
- Level 3 (tertiary) – resources and allocations.

This method of thinking has particular attraction and relevance to the delivery of healthcare and therefore the educational need to aid that delivery.

Level 1 addresses the needs of those for whom the system ultimately exists, that is, patients.

Level 2 addresses the needs of service-providers, who have a direct relationship to those in Level 1. They also provide information, services or training that will affect others in Level 2. The interesting parallel with educational needs assessment for doctors is that those at Level 2 (service-providers) may also have unmet needs related to the functions they perform in relation either to their colleagues (Level 2) or to patients (Level 1).

Level 3 considers the needs of the organisation as an organisation. In terms of general practice education, this could be viewed as the role of the Department of Postgraduate Medical and Dental Education (PGMDE) or the workforce development confederations (WDCs). Both have a role in identifying and allocating resources to meet the needs of service development and, ultimately, the care of patients.

The government is not only committed to needs assessment for continuing professional development but also for the delivery of healthcare. In the summer of 1997 the then newly elected Labour government declared its intention to 'secure equal access to services for all the population on the basis of clinical need' (DoH, 1997).

A health service based on needs relies on needs assessment to influence the allocation of resources. Effective health needs assessment on the practice or local population should enable primary care trusts to make informed decisions about the allocation of valuable resources.

For example, a practice which serves a high Asian population may identify a high prevalence of diabetes. This could highlight the need for increased diabetic care and an improved knowledge of those undertaking the care of this specific group of patients. The educational need may be met by allowing various members of the team to undertake a course in diabetic care.

Although population needs assessment must take account of many factors, including epidemiological research and local social and environmental issues, many of the assessment tools described earlier in this chapter will be a useful starting point for GPs and their practice teams.

Educational needs assessment and healthcare needs assessment must be considered in relation to:

- the healthcare needs of individual patients
- the healthcare needs of the practice population
- the healthcare needs of the community
- the educational needs of GPs
- the educational needs of other team members
- the educational needs of the organisation.

Setting priorities and influencing the educational programme

No matter how good the use of the tools, there is little point in applying them if the outcome is not translated into some kind of action. Understanding the healthcare needs of the practice population can help to deploy limited resources more efficiently. Knowing what patients need collectively, and when they need it, can make for better use of time. We can then consider how the existing skills within the practice team match up to those patient needs. If there are considerable discrepancies it might be necessary to train individuals to be competent in these areas. It is at this stage that we may find tension between the educational needs of individuals and the educational needs of the organisation.

For example, a practice nurse may wish to undertake a diploma in family planning, but the perceived organisational need is for the nurse to undertake a diploma in CHD. A GP may wish to undertake a course in acupuncture but the perceived organisational need is for GPs to develop their skills in joint injections. Meeting the organisational need does not necessarily preclude meeting individuals' needs. The practice and the individual will have to negotiate levels of priority.

There is not necessarily always conflict between organisational and individual learning needs. Organisational needs will, on occasions, provide individuals with opportunities that they perhaps did not know existed or had not previously considered. Individuals may then adapt their learning needs to meet the needs of the organisation.

For example, a primary care organisation may want to develop GPs with special interests (GPwSI). As an organisation, it will identify what the need is and specify exactly what is wanted. This may appeal to a GP currently employed as a clinical assistant in that speciality who may have been previously unaware of this opportunity. The GP may now choose to facilitate her development and learning needs to meet the needs of the primary care organisation in this new role.

Inevitably, at times there will be tensions for all doctors in addressing their personal educational needs and the needs of the practice. There may also be tension when prioritising the pursuit of learning for an identified need and learning for something that is of particular interest. The *Good CPD Guide* (Grant *et al.*, 1999) acknowledges the notion that, given a choice, doctors will focus their learning on things with which they are already familiar and are interested in rather than selecting more challenging areas that are new to them. Although it also states that evidence for such statements is rarely available, the concept may well be linked to the failure of doctors to have fully grasped the needs assessment process (Myers, 1999). There is absolutely nothing wrong with developing knowledge on topics which are of particular interest. However, the problem comes if this is done at the expense of those things that need to be learnt to fill knowledge or skills gaps. When confronted by the decision as to whether to learn something of particular interest or something that is an identified need, we need to ask the following question.

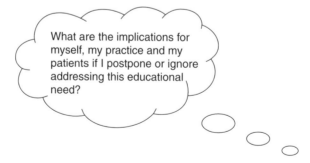

What are the implications for myself, my practice and my patients if I postpone or ignore addressing this educational need?

The learning needs of doctors and their teams should not only influence resource allocation for healthcare. They should also influence those involved in planning education and training. This is equally true of HPE and continuing professional development.

There is little evidence to show that the postgraduate education allowance (PGEA), introduced in 1990, either addressed GPs' needs or formed part of a planned education programme or curriculum (Tracey *et al.*, 1997). The introduction of personal development plans and practice professional development plans is encouraging a move away from such ad hoc learning towards planning learning for individuals and for practices (Gallen and Buckle, 2001). However, these plans are only useful if based on some form of educational needs assessment. Identification of educational needs should influence education programmes. GP tutors, continuing professional development tutors, primary care tutors and the education leads from primary care organisations are charged with the provision of postgraduate education for GPs and their primary healthcare teams. In order for this provision and facilitation to be part of a meaningful educational strategy it must be based on educational needs assessment, not ad hoc learning.

Summary

- Educational needs assessment is used by medical educators to mean the process by which learners' educational needs are identified or diagnosed.
- There are many methods of educational needs assessment. No one method is necessarily better than another. The best method is that which is appropriate and relevant to learners.
- Educational needs assessment should take account of the healthcare needs of the practice population.
- There may be tensions between individual learning needs and organisational learning needs.
- There is a place for opportunistic learning and learning for interest rather than identified need. However, the importance of striking a balance between this and needs-directed learning should not be underestimated.

- Educational needs assessment should inform educational planning strategies and curriculum development.

References

Bogdan R and Bilken S (1992) *Qualitative Research for Education: an introduction to theory and methods* (2e). Allyn & Bacon, Needham Heights, MA.

Bradshaw J (1972) A taxonomy of social need. In: A McLachlan (ed.) *Problems and Progress in Medical Care* (7 series). OUP, London.

Department of Health (1997) *The New NHS: modern, dependable.* The Stationery Office, London.

Department of Health (2001) *Working Together – Learning Together. A framework for lifelong learning.* The Stationery Office, London.

Eve R (2000) Learning with PUNs and DENs: a method for determining educational needs and the evaluation of its use in primary care. *Education in General Practice* **11**, 73–79.

Gallen D and Buckle G (2001) *Personal and Practice Development Plans in Primary Care: a guide to getting started.* Butterworth Heinemann, Oxford.

Grant J (2002) Learning needs assessment: assessing the need. *British Medical Journal* **334**, 156–159.

Grant J, Chambers R and Jackson G (eds) (1999) *Good CPD Guide.* Reed Healthcare, Sutton.

Mann K (1998) Not another survey. Using questionnaires effectively in needs assessment. *Journal of Continuing Education in the Health Profession* **18**, 142–149.

Myers P (1999) The objective assessment of general practitioners' educational needs: an under-researched area? *British Journal of General Practice* **49**, 303–307.

Servier R (1989) Conducting focus group research. *Journal of College Admissions* **122**, 4–9.

Stritter F, Tresolini C and Reeb K (1994) The Delphi technique in curriculum development. *Teaching and Learning in Medicine* **6**, 136–141.

Stroebe W and Diehl M (1994) Why groups are less effective than their members: on productivity losses in idea generating groups. In: W Stroebe and M Hewstone (eds) *European Review of Social Psychology*. John Wiley and Sons, Chichester.

Tracey J, Arroll B, Barham P and Richmond D (1997) The validity of general practitioner self assessment of knowledge: cross sectional study. *British Medical Journal* 315, 1426–1428.

Witkin B (1995) *Planning and Conducting Needs Assessment: a practical guide*. Sage Publications, London.

5

Fit for purpose: continuing professional development

Introduction

This chapter looks at the concept of life-long learning and the distinction between continuous medical education and continuing professional development. It considers the tools that will be needed to facilitate the change to life-long learning and the role of the HPE tutor in delivering life-long learners.

Can you describe the difference between CME and CPD? What are the main differences?

The current situation

Over the last few years there has been a great change in emphasis of continuous education for health professionals. The Chief Medical Officer's review of GP education has set in place a shift in focus from continuous medical education to continuing professional development for all health professionals (Calman, 1998). The reasons for this are clear when it is considered that continuous medical education for GPs has largely failed in its remit to produce both quality and relevance to education. Instead, it has focused on the quantity of courses attended (DoH, 1998a; Field, 1998; Boulay, 2000). Indeed, evidence for reflective learning is limited and few studies actually show change in clinical behaviour after educational events (Berg, 1979; Haynes *et al.*, 1984; Davis *et al.*, 1992). This may, in part, be due to the method of the introduction of the new contract in 1990. GPs had their seniority allowances reduced and their vocational training allowance scrapped to pay for attendance at educational meetings. In order to earn back the salary reduction, doctors had to attend 30 hours per year of educational sessions to claim the postgraduate education allowance (PGEA). Attendance is optional; payments are a reward for attending a minimum of six hours on a rising scale to 30 hours. Although the government originally created this allowance as a grant, with which GPs could purchase high-quality education, Pitts *et al.* (1999) showed that it was regarded as 'stolen money' by the profession. Education therefore was achieved as cheaply as possibly and usually followed a non-interactive lecture format (Pitts, 1993).

Thus the PGEA is restricted to principals in general practice. It disenfranchised a growing number of non-principals who are not eligible for it. It also tended to be uniprofessional in focus (Field, 1998). The low educational value and failure to change professional practice of much continuous medical education has inevitably led to criticism of its emphasis on formal didactic teaching and academic knowledge. The links between theory and practice in professional work and its effectiveness have proved difficult to evaluate (Brigley *et al.*, 1997).

Although GPs value educational activities in their professional development, these were assigned a relatively small role in bringing about specific changes in clinical behaviour (Drage *et al.*, 1994).

The then Chief Medical Officer was clearly aware of the principles of self-directed adult learning as described by Brookfield (1986). Calman (1998) placed them within the overall context of integrated multidisciplinary education for the whole health service. The purpose of his review was to produce improved patient care underpinned by evidence and a valued process of development. The principal proposal was to integrate and improve the educational process through a 'practice professional developmental plan' (PPDP). Plans developed at practice level could allow accurate assessment of the needs of practitioners, patients and all staff by use of existing practice strengths and resources. They could build on current strategies and systems in the least threatening environment (Houghton and Wall, 1999).

The shift to PPDPs is based on the following:

* formal needs assessment
* practice-based learning in the areas identified by those involved
* the potential (if not compunction) for multidisciplinary learning.

Strategy for starting a PPDP

A practice can use protected learning time (time when the practice is shut and cover is provided by the local co-operative) to focus on the health needs of its population. All members of the primary healthcare team can make a contribution. The practice may identify that it has a high rate of teenage pregnancies and seek to offer a more teenage-sensitive service. This would include everyone from receptionist to practice nurse and doctors being more aware of the needs and sensitivities of this group of teenagers by perhaps offering drop-in clinics during school lunch breaks.

The distinction between continuous medical education and continuing professional development

Brigley *et al.* (1997) described HPE for medical professionals as:

- de-personalised
- de-contextualised
- learning-fragmented and individualistic
- knowledge impermeable, owned by professional élites and closed to non-professionals.

In this description Brigley *et al.* (1997) raise some critical questions about the implied relationship between professional development and academic knowledge in medical education. With the question of whether academic knowledge of medicine can be learnt apart from the context in which it is applied, these authors also raised the issue of how the relationship between practice and theory may be cemented in professional studies – both initial and continuing.

Continuous medical education – which is focused now only on individual doctors and their scientific and technological upgrading – blindly assumes that qualified and up-to-date medical professionals can intuitively match specialist knowledge to the demands of actual cases. The principal focus of continuous medical education is on individuals' professions and their perceived knowledge gap related to their professional work. In contrast, Brigley *et al.* (1997) emphasised that continuing professional development is:

- self-directed learning
- professional self-awareness
- learning developed in context
- multidisciplinary and multilevel collaboration
- the learning needs of individuals and their organisations
- an enquiry-based concept of professionalism.

It also involves widening accountability to patients, the community, managers and policy-makers, providing a form of evaluation that is integral, participatory and collaborative rather than externally driven.

Some university medical schools (notably that of McMaster in Canada, Maastricht in the Netherlands and Newcastle in Australia) have begun to recast the link between academic knowledge and effective practice. They aim to develop the learning of scientific knowledge through clinical experience, problem-solving and practice-based work. This challenge to the separation of theory and practice in learning is premised on the view that specialist academic knowledge only becomes professional knowledge when it is applied practically in a particular clinical context.

Where problem-based learning has been adopted as the mainstay of the curriculum, its application is expected to fulfil two quite distinct purposes. One aim is to use problem-based learning as a method that will assist students towards achieving a specific set of objectives, to become capable in a set of competences that will be important to them throughout their professional life.

For example, a doctor might seek to gain better skills in dealing with aggressive patients. This could be undertaken by the use of actors to pose as aggressive patients and allowing the doctor to practise various techniques or approaches that might help the situation.

The second aim is to use problem-based learning as the method of choice because it is particularly suitable to support the conditions that influence effective adult learning (Engel, 1997).

For example, learners learn best when they can relate the knowledge to their day-to-day activities. So discussing the problems of treating a patient with diabetes that the doctor knows is more powerful than just a discussion of diabetes.

Getting doctors to understand the significance of life-long learning

The development of PPDPs should be in conjunction with individuals' personal development plans that Calman (1998) emphasised that all health professionals must have by 1 April 2000. Individuals' development of personal development plans is crucial to the thinking that now underpins the education agenda (Towle, 1998). Individuals have to identify their own learning needs in conjunction with those of the organisation within which they work. In the immediate instance this will be the primary care setting but also already includes the NHS as the umbrella organisation. The various levels of needs assessment have already been discussed in Chapter 4 (p. 77). There is, therefore, an interplay between Level 1, those for whom the services are provided, and Level 3, which provides the full infrastructure but does not see service provision on an individual basis. This is where the dilemma with regard to educational needs assessment lies and is the driving force behind competing agendas. Morrison and Spencer (1999) suggest that as the service needs of general practice continue to increase there may be even less time available in the future to address educational needs and to seek support from colleagues who themselves have less time.

This means that the protected time offered by HPE in the first year after vocational training is an essential element in the continuing professional development of individual doctors. The facility to have protected locum cover time of 20 days per year allows for a more structured and focused educational programme to be developed by individuals. It gives them time to attend courses but, more specifically, time for reflection and critically evaluating their own educational wants and needs.

Doctors will have to consider the agendas of:

• clinical governance
• revalidation

- national service frameworks
- health improvement programmes
- the National Institute for Clinical Excellence (NICE).

These all create a workload imposed from government that health professionals need to respond to whilst developing themselves and their practices.

The draft consultation document from the Royal College of General Practitioners (RCGP) and the General Practitioners Committee (GPC) entitled *Good Medical Practice for General Practitioners* (RCGP/GPC, 1999) outlines the standards required for being a good doctor.

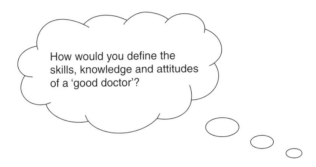

How would you define the skills, knowledge and attitudes of a 'good doctor'?

This document forms the basis both of the appraisal process and the revalidation process and needs to be read and understood by all GPs. Again, the significance of continuing professional development, as opposed to continuous medical education, is highlighted. For example, excellent GPs:

- are up-to-date with developments in clinical practice and regularly review their knowledge and performance
- use these reviews to develop practice and personal developmental plans
- use a range of methods to monitor different aspects of care and to meet their educational needs.

This places the emphasis very much on a bottom-up approach to educational needs assessment by individuals, as discussed in Chapter 4, who can then feed them into the PPDP, the local agenda through primary care groups and the national agenda of the Department of Health.

Continuing professional development has been described by Madden and Mitchell (1993) as 'the maintenance and enhancement of the knowledge, expertise and confidence of the professional throughout their career according to a plan formulated with regard to the need of the professional, the employer and the professional society'.

Although updating and enhancement has inevitably been a feature of many professional careers for far longer, continuing professional development as a concept was relatively unknown until at least the 1960s (Houle, 1980). Only in the last 10–15 years have professional bodies taken systematic steps to ensure that their members continue their development on an ongoing basis. The inadequacy of initial professional education as a preparation for an entire working life is now well-recognised by professional bodies. It was this recognition that enabled HPE to take a place on the national agenda, as the need for further development of the vocational training scheme has been recognised for some time. It is not just that knowledge dates, but that the very concept and interpretation of professional tasks and roles changes over time (Gear *et al.*, 1994). The increasing numbers of doctors having a 'portfolio career' (in which doctors have several different jobs and responsibilities, not just standard GMS) will have to ensure that they are up-to-date at each aspect of their career portfolio.

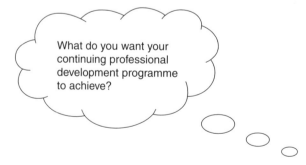

What do you want your continuing professional development programme to achieve?

Within the definition of continuing professional development we can identify different ways in which educational needs assessment should be approached in healthcare:

> 'Continual Professional Development is a process of life-long learning for all individuals and teams which meet the needs of patients and deliver the health outcomes and health priorities of the NHS and which enables professionals to expand and to fulfil their potential.' (*A First Class Service*, DoH, 1998a)

Continuing professional development programmes need to meet both the following:

* the learning needs of health professionals to inspire public confidence in their skills
* the learning needs to meet the wider service development needs of the NHS (Calman, 1998).

The significance, therefore, of life-long learning is the continued development of individuals, as professionals within the wider context of the health needs of both the practice population and the wider NHS. This development could never be fulfilled by a continuous medical education programme which by its very nature is a disjointed selection of educational events that have not undergone any formal educational evaluation.

Developing life-long learning

The identification of learning needs is the crucial first step towards formal thinking about continuing professional development. It can help make implicit methods explicit, 'to change haphazard approaches into systematic ones and to replace the ad hoc with the planned response' (Brigley *et al.*, 1997).

The report of the Chief Medical Officer on continuing professional development in general practice (May 1998) highlighted that for all health organisations the core principles are that continuing professional development should:

- be targeted
- identify education needs
- be educationally effective
- have some form of needs assessment to precede the development of the programme
- become mandatory.

It is also essential that we look to ensure that any new HPE programme does not fall into the trap of the ad hoc lecture-style format, but is properly needs assessed for the individuals concerned in relation to the wider health agenda.

Remedial learning

A First Class Service (DoH, 1998a) sets out a model for a continuing professional development cycle (with the first part of the cycle being the 'assessment of individual and organisational needs' – again highlighting the link between needs assessment and continuing professional development). Needs assessment is the only way by which factors such as knowledge, skills, competence and habits, which detract from ultimate performance, may be dissected to reveal specific deficiencies. It is this aspect of educational needs assessment that has been used to explore the gaps in individuals' knowledge bases and thereby identify methods of moving individuals forward. If introduced sensitively, needs assessment could be the way by which recalcitrant individuals may be convinced of the need for continual learning (Ward, 1988). Although remedial training is not the preserve of HPE programmes, both are concerned with the recognition of knowledge gaps and allowing individuals the means to undertake further study.

Example of the effect of needs assessment and the delivery of continuing professional development

Rosendaal *et al.* (1994) showed how course content was improved through multiple methods of needs assessment. These authors used a multifaceted approach to needs assessment when planning and implementing a short continuous medical education programme in gastroenterology. Pre-course questionnaires, focus groups and individual interviews were used to form the course content. There is a move in primary care to relate the provision of continuing professional education to the educational needs of participants, as in the model of individual portfolio-based learning (RCGP, 1993) and Myers (1999). These portfolios may also be used in the appraisal and revalidation process. It therefore becomes essential that doctors on the vocational training scheme should be developing their personal development plans or portfolio, and should use the appraisal process to look at their individual needs for continuing professional development.

Educational needs and continuing professional development are real and intertwined, in that effective continuing professional development must begin with an evaluation of the needs of individuals or organisations. This will enable a clearer plan to emerge of the programme to be undertaken to meet needs already identified.

HPE is just a single year in practitioners' continuing professional development, but allows individuals to focus on areas relevant to themselves and their practice.

How will a HPE tutor then develop a curriculum for the needs of newly qualified doctors?

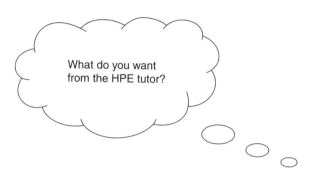

What do you want from the HPE tutor?

HPE tutors should consider themselves as facilitators of educational programmes. They should have the skills to:

- undertake educational needs assessments for individuals or within the group setting
- offer advice
- facilitate educational needs
- support HPE learners.

The question of when these tasks should be undertaken is clearly very important. If individuals are to maximise their learning opportunities within the framework of HPE then they should be planning their programmes whilst they are still on vocational training schemes. HPE tutors could liaise with the vocational training scheme course organisers both by informing registrars of the programme and by helping to structure programmes for individuals. Needs assessment could therefore be conducted during the vocational training scheme (albeit towards the end) and take into account what both course organisers and HPE trainers have also identified as either gaps in knowledge or curricula.

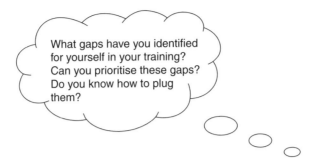

The literature has already given clues as to areas in which GP registrars feel ill-equipped or lacking in knowledge at the end of their vocational training. This information may be used as a basis to help kick-start the HPE programme. HPE tutors could send questionnaires to those joining the scheme or, indeed, run focus groups (as discussed in Chapter 2). The point of the educational needs assessment in this group is not that HPE tutors may then provide a series of ad hoc lectures, which purport to fulfil needs that individuals have already stated; rather, HPE tutors need to be able to offer a wide range of solutions to those educational needs, covering the whole gamut from:

- a simple lecture
- interactive workshops
- attendance at clinics
- personal reading, to
- experiential learning
- visiting 'beacon' practices
- mentoring
- educational project work.

Fit for purpose

The NHS Plan (DoH, 2000) calls itself an ambitious but practical blueprint to restore and modernise the health service.

It also highlights areas that will need major educational input to ensure its success. The following are just some examples.

- Primary care will provide a greater range of services.
- Successful, flexible, multidisciplinary working with respect for individual professionals will be developed further to deliver better services to patients.
- All GPs to have access to NHSnet.
- A thousand GP specialists (GPs with special interests).

These goals will need a co-ordinated approach across all health professionals and incorporation into continuing professional development programmes if they are to be realised.

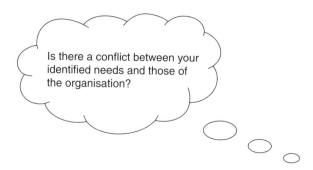

In essence, *The NHS Plan* (DoH, 2000), as outlined above and including *The New NHS: modern, dependable* (DoH, 1997) and *Our Healthier Nation* (DoH, 1998b), has an agenda that could be viewed in complete isolation of individuals' own perceptions of their educational needs. The NHS has to deliver *The NHS Plan* (DoH, 2000) and this can add to the dilemma of individuals who rather than undertake any personal needs assessments just conform to the needs of the organisation. Tension arises from the fact that individuals may choose to do only what they want and be of no help to the national agenda, or may only want what they must do for the national agenda at the expense of their own development. The PPDP should be capable of marrying these conflicting agendas. Individuals will have input into the PPDP, and the contents of their own personal development plans will inform the practice plan. Practices may then also take account of national imperatives, such as national service frameworks, and tailor their delivery to the skills of the primary healthcare team. That said, we do need to use the time available during professional education to produce doctors that are fit for purpose in the new NHS. This will involve them in learning skills and becoming more knowledgeable in areas of clinical care and management.

HPE time could be used to develop the skills and knowledge necessary for GP specialisation (GPs with special interests) that *The NHS Plan* (DoH, 2000) is actually demanding. Clearly, there is no time on the current vocational training scheme to fully develop these skills and, indeed, the time available for HPE may only just start the process.

Summary

- The PGEA will be replaced.
- Continuous medical education does not fulfil the needs of continuing professional development.
- There remains tension between the needs of individuals and the needs of organisations.
- The key to development remains the personal and practice developmental plans.
- *Good Medical Practice for General Practitioners* (RCGP/GPC, 1999) is a key document in the appraisal or revalidation process.
- The profession needs to understand and help deliver *The NHS Plan* (DoH, 2000).
- The role of HPE tutors is that of facilitators.
- We need to produce doctors that are 'fit for purpose' in the new NHS.

References

Berg AO (1979) Does continuing medical education improve the quality of medical care? A look at the evidence. *Journal of Family Practice* **8**, 1171–1174.

Boulay C (2000) From CME to CPD: getting better at getting better? *British Medical Journal* **320**, 393–394.

Brigley S, Young Y, Littlejohns P and McEwen J (1997) Continuing education for medical professionals: a reflective model. *Postgraduate Medical Journal* **73**, 23–26.

Brookfield SD (1986) *Understanding and Facilitating Adult Learning*. Open University Press, Milton Keynes.

Calman K (1998) *A Review of Continuing Professional Development in General Practice*. Department of Health, London.

Davis DA, Thomson MA, Oxman AD and Haynes RB (1992) Evidence for the effectiveness of CME. A review of 50 randomized trials. *JAMA* **268**, 1111–1117.

Department of Health (1997) *The New NHS: modern, dependable*. DoH, London.

Department of Health (1998a) *A First Class Service: quality in the new NHS*. DoH, London.

Department of Health (1998b) *Our Healthier Nation: a contract for health*. DoH, London.

Department of Health (2000) *The NHS Plan: the Government's response to the Royal Commission on long-term care*. DoH, London.

Drage M, Wakeford R and Wharton A (1994) What do general practitioners think changes their clinical behaviour? *Education for General Practice* **5**, 48–53.

Engel CE (1997) Not just a method but a way of learning. In: D Boud and G Feletti (eds) *The Challenge of Problem Based Learning* (2e). Kogan Page, London.

Field S (1998) The Chief Medical Officer's review of continuing professional development: the end to the PGEA system. *Education in General Practice* **9**, 299–301.

Gear J, McIntosh A and Squires G (1994) *Informal Learning in the Professions*. University of Hull, Department of Adult Education.

Haynes RB, Davis D, McKibbon A and Tugwell P (1984) A critical appraisal of the efficacy of continuing medical education. *JAMA* **251**, 61–64.

Houghton G and Wall D (1999) Clinical governance and the Chief Medical Officer's review of GP education: piecing the new NHS jigsaw together. *Medical Teacher* **21**, 5–6.

Houle CO (1980) *Continuing Learning in the Professions*. Jossey-Bass, San Francisco, CA.

Madden CA and Mitchell VA (1993) *Professions, Standards and Competence: a survey of continuing education for the professions*. Department for Continuing Education, University of Bristol.

Morrison J and Spencer J (1999) Educational needs after completion of vocational training in general practice. *Medical Education* **33**, 790–791.

Myers P (1999) The objective assessment of general practitioners' educational needs: an under researched area? *British Journal of General Practice* **49**, 303–307.

Pitts J (1993) 'Making allowances' – use of and attitudes towards the postgraduate education allowance. *Postgraduate Education in General Practice* **4**, 198–202.

Pitts J, Curtis A, While R and Holloway I (1999) Practice professional developmental plans: general practitioners' perspectives on proposed changes in general practice education. *British Journal of General Practice* **49**, 959–962.

Rosendaal GM, Lockyer JM and Sutherland LR (1994) Improving course content through multiple methods of needs assessment: a demonstration project. *Teaching and Learning in Medicine* **6**, 269–273.

Royal College of General Practitioners (RCGP) (1993) *Portfolio-based Learning in General Practice* (Occasional Paper 63). Royal College of General Practitioners, London.

Royal College of General Practitioners (RCGP) and General Practitioners' Committee (GPC) (1999) *Good Medical Practice for General Practitioners*. Draft document for consultation. Royal College of General Practitioners, London.

Towle A (1998) Changes in health care and continuing medical education for the 21st century. *British Medical Journal* **316**, 301–304.

Ward J (1988) Continuing medical education. Part 2. Needs assessment in continuing medical education. *Medical Journal of Australia* **148**, 77–80.

Further reading

Department of Health (DoH) (2000) *National Service Framework for Cardiovascular Disease*. Department of Health, London.

Department of Health (DoH) (2000) *National Service Framework for Mental Health*. Department of Health, London.

Myers P and Mahmood K (1997) Key facts as an aid to developing CME for general practitioners. *Education for General Practice* **8**, 238–241.

Osbourne C, Davies J and Garnett J (1998) Guiding the student to the centre of the stakeholder curriculum: independent and work-based learning at Middlesex University. In: J Stephenson and M Yorke (eds) *Capability and Quality in Higher Education*. Kogan Page, London.

Peach L (1998) Individual and organisational learning. *Journal of Continuing Professional Development* **1**, 11–15.

Peck C, McCall M, McLaren B and Rotem T (2000) Continuing medical education and continuing professional development: international comparisons. *British Medical Journal* **320**, 432–435.

Pell J and Williams S (1999) Do nursing home residents make greater demands on GPs? A prospective comparative study. *British Journal of General Practice* **49**, 527–530.

Pendleton D (1995) Professional development in primary care: problems, puzzles and paradigms. *British Journal of General Practice* **45**, 377–381.

Pereles L and Russell ML (1996) Needs for CME in geriatrics. Part 1. Perceptions of patients and community informants. *Canadian Family Physician* **42**, 437–445.

Pereles L and Russell ML (1996) Needs for CME in geriatrics. Part 2. Physician priorities and perceptions of community representatives. *Canadian Family Physician* **42**, 632–640.

6

Curriculum planning

Introduction

This chapter seeks to highlight the concept of a curriculum as it pertains to HPE. We will outline both methods and templates to aid learners in adopting a systematic approach to planning their year. Reference will be made to adult learning theory and professional development plans, and also to adult learning styles. It is important for learners to grasp the best method of learning for themselves. They need to understand that the curriculum is just like a menu and that they need to choose what they want and need from that menu. It can be quite counterproductive to attend didactic lectures if the preferred learning style is that of an activist (one of the learning styles, see later). Although this chapter is not intended to be a list of educational topics that may or may not pertain to HPE, we will make reference to the literature that has suggested areas or knowledge gaps that those entering general practice for the first time have highlighted.

The curriculum

It is impossible to get everything in medical education fitted into a limited timescale. Trainers on the Kettering vocational training scheme tried to look at the contents of a core curriculum for the GP registrar year on a study day. It was clear by the end of the day that the 'core' elements (as defined by the group) would have taken 18 months to complete. An impossible task!

There are many ways of defining a curriculum. An exact definition of *curriculum* may be elusive. A curriculum is more than any one of the following.

* A plan that will determine an education experience.
* A timetable.
* A list of contents.
* A list of objectives.
* A list of learning experiences.
* Even students that are getting together for the purpose of fulfilling the course objective.

One of the best definitions of a *curriculum* that has been proposed is, 'Everything that happens in relation to the educational programme'.

The advantage of this definition is that it encompasses many different aspects of the curriculum.

* The *formal* (everything that is intended to be included).
* The *informal* curriculum (what can be learnt just from interaction on the course).
* The *hidden* curriculum (what students learn that the course has not specifically tried to teach).
* The *null* curriculum (what the course is not trying to teach, for example doctors who make errors).

It encompasses learning arising from a wide range of educational strategies, such as student-centred learning, community-based education and task-based learning.

The real problem for HPE students is the narrow thinking that may occur in relation to trying to develop a curriculum for their year. One immediately thinks of a form of curriculum or list of topics that students have to 'get through' within an allotted timespan. Unfortunately, this totally negates the experiential learning that will occur throughout the year, which may ultim-ately be of greater benefit than any of the formal curriculum that students have devised.

Consider Figure 6.1, developed by Honey and Mumford (1986), which represents individuals' learning.

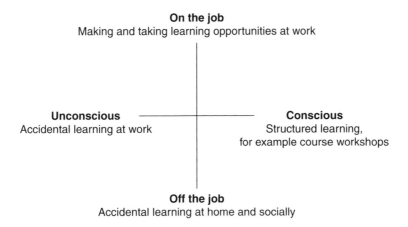

Figure 6.1: How individuals learn.

Figure 6.1 amply demonstrates the importance and range of learning activities that occur outside of what could be con-sidered a formal curriculum. It is therefore worth emphasising that individuals embarking on HPE should understand the range of opportunities that are available to them rather than constrain their thinking to simple course work.

Learning styles

Understanding of the importance of learning approaches has been sharpened by Entwhistle and Ramsden (1983). These authors categorised learning approaches as deep, surface and strategic. To each learning approach there correspond differ-ences in students' motivation and strategy.

- Deep learners aim to achieve understanding.

- Surface learners tend only to meet the task requirement.
- Strategic learners look to achieve the best results from a given input.

One of the major problems of continuing professional development is how to transform the surface approach of learning into a deep learning strategy. Perry (1981) emphasised the importance of this shift from superficial to deep learning as a method of building on existing knowledge. He showed that learners using this approach are more likely to retain knowledge and to think strategically.

HPE does not have any assessment processes. Formal examinations still tend to be the focus of a year's teaching and encourage superficial learning. Indeed, the assessment process tends to drive the curriculum, as has already been experienced in medical school and during the vocational training scheme. Since there is no assessment process in life-long learning, the curriculum must be driven by other modalities. The aim is to develop the deeper learning style and not to have a superficial approach to the educational content of the subject matter. Individuals who find the best method of learning for themselves will clearly help the development of deep learning during this year.

Learning styles may be a combination of cognitive, affective and physical factors, which display how learners process, interact with and relate to a learning environment. Cognitive factors are those pertaining to the learning process itself; affective factors relate to the feelings, expectation and motivation towards learning, whereas physical factors refer to students' reactions to their surroundings.

For example, breaking bad news is a task that can encompass all three of the above. You need to have the communication skills to undertake the task, an understanding of the effect what you will say will have on the person and yourself. Lastly, you need to find the right environment to undertake the task. The middle of the waiting room is not the best place for this!

In Valley (1997) the term 'learning style' indicates, for instance, 'the preference that an individual may have for processing information in a particular way when coming out of learning activity. Learning styles involve the cognitive processes that are implicated in learning; they can be thought of as habits that allow a learner to benefit more from some experiences than from others'.

One of the most common learning style questionnaires remains that of Honey and Mumford (1986) which measures an individual's tendency towards a particular learning style. These are activist, reflector, theorist and pragmatist.

Activists

Activists involve themselves fully and without bias in new experiences. They enjoy the 'here and now' and are happy to be dominated by immediate experiences. They are open-minded, not sceptical and this tends to make them enthusiastic about anything new. Their philosophy is 'I'll try anything once.' They tend to act first and consider the consequences afterwards. Their days are filled with activity. They tackle problems by brainstorming. As soon as the excitement from one activity has died down they are busy looking for the next. They tend to thrive on the challenge of new experiences, but are bored with implementation and long-term consolidation. They are gregarious people, constantly involving themselves with others, but in so doing they seek to centre all activities on themselves.

Reflectors

Reflectors like to stand back to ponder experiences and observe them from many perspectives. They collect data, both first-hand and from others, and prefer to think about it thoroughly before coming to any conclusion. The thorough collection and analysis of data about experience and events is what counts so they tend to postpone reaching definitive conclusions for as long as possible. Their philosophy is to be cautious. They are thoughtful people who like to consider all possible angles and implications before making a move. They prefer to take a back seat in meetings and discussions; they enjoy observing other people in action. They listen to others and get the drift of the discussion before making their own points. They tend to adopt a low profile and have a slightly distant, tolerant, unruffled air about them. When they act it is part of the wider picture which includes the past as well as the present, and others' observations as well as their own.

Theorists

Theorists are direct and integrate observations into complex but logically sounded theories. They think problems through in a vertical step-by-step logical way. They assimilate disparate facts into coherent theories. They tend to be perfectionists who will not rest easily until they fit into a rational scheme. They like to analyse and synthesise. They are keen on basic assumptions, principles, theory models and system thinking. Their philosophy prizes rationality and logic. If it is logical it is good. Questions they ask frequently are, 'Does it make sense?', 'How does this fit with that?' and 'What are the basic assumptions?' They tend to be detached, analytical and dedicated to rational objectivity rather than anything subjective or ambiguous. Their approach to problems is consistently logical. This is their mental set and they rigidly reject anything that does not fit with it. They prefer to maximise certainty and feel uncomfortable with subjective judgements, lateral thinking and anything flippant.

Pragmatists

Pragmatists are keen on trying out new ideas, theories and techniques to see if they work in practice. They positively search out new ideas and take the first opportunity to experiment with applications. They are the sort of people who return from management courses brimming with new ideas that they want to try out in practice. They like to get on with things and act quickly and confidently on ideas that attract them. They tend to be impatient with ruminating and open-ended discussion. They are essentially practical, down-to-earth people who like making practical decisions and solving problems. They respond to problems and opportunities as a challenge. Their philosophy is 'There's always a better way' and 'If it works it's good.'

Although there are certainly other learning styles and questionnaires than that of Honey and Mumford, theirs is a very simple tool for identifying your own preferred learning style. Its strength lies in not just undertaking the questionnaire once, but in repeating the questionnaire at some point later on during the year to see if your preferred style has changed.

It has been well documented that those entering vocational training schemes have a very activist pragmatic style at the start of the registrar year and that this moves some way towards a more reflective theorist style by the end of that year.

Agenda

If learners now have an understanding of their preferred learning styles, this will help them to develop their own agendas for the HPE year.

A study by the Joint Committee for Education (JCE, 1998) showed that whilst there is a vast range of types of educational provision available, the first year after the vocational training scheme is a period of significant unmet need. Young doctors have a tendency to learn about clinical topics but were also not satisfied by the topics covered. They were learning in a haphazard way and often in isolation. Contact with peers was considered very important and distance learning was not favoured at all. The preferred method of learning, according to the study (JCE, 1998), was short lectures, with opportunities for interaction.

It is interesting to note that the learning topics recommended by more than 50% of those questioned were:

- practice management and organisation
- clinical development or consolidation
- financial management in practice
- personal educational planning.

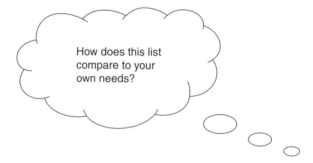

How does this list compare to your own needs?

The Joint Committee for Education study (1998) was undertaken before the publication of the Calman paper on continuing professional development (Calman, 1998) that highlighted the need for personal and practice developmental plans. It would therefore not be unexpected that one of the needs of young doctors would be the development of personal development plans. Accepting this need would assist in fulfilling the other recommendations of the report, namely, the need to have a more strategic approach to education and to achieve seamless training rather than the current disjointed series of stages at present. We need to co-ordinate the methods of learning, needs assessment, integration with practice and assessment of outcomes at each stage if this is to be achieved.

Personal planning

What then are the first steps in planning the HPE year?

It may help to ask four key questions and to write short notes or ideas down on a piece of paper. Do not be daunted by the task and try to focus on areas of real need. The four questions form the backbone of the personal development plan and are:

1 Where am I now?
2 Where do I want to be?
3 What tools will I use to get there?
4 How can I demonstrate that I have achieved my goal?

The original list may be long but it can be honed down into a more manageable and workable list by also considering the following.

- What are the needs of the practice within which I work?
- What are the needs of the patient population?
- What are the local morbidity and mortality rates?
- What levels of deprivation are encountered locally?
- What educational opportunities exist within the locality?
- What areas of the 'Good Doctor Guide' do I still need to work on?

Cross-referencing the answers to the original list may help to sort out the priority areas for the coming year. Remember, do not attempt to solve all your educational needs, as it can be discouraging to keep looking at a long list of needs that remain unfulfilled. Continuing professional development tutors, or indeed those tutors who have a specific remit to work on HPE, may well be worth engaging to help to focus efforts.

Tools to help

It can be difficult to know what you do not know, but there are many tools to help in this quest.

Patients' unmet needs (PUNs) and doctors' educational needs (DENs)

As already discussed in Chapter 4, this is a useful method of identifying doctors' needs in relation to the needs of the patients they see in surgery. Eve (1994, 2000) introduced this method. After seeing patients in surgery he wrote down what unmet needs they had in that consultation and then thought about what educational needs this highlighted for himself.

Typically, doctors have a sheet of paper besides them in the surgery and they jot down points, arising from consultations, that patients wanted to know but that doctors did not necessarily have answers for at that time. At the end of the surgery doctors could reflect on the main points highlighted and perhaps focus on those that had arisen more than once in the session. The great value of the PUNs and DENs method is that it is work-based experiential learning and very relevant to doctors' (and patients') day-to-day needs.

Significant event analysis

This has also been called 'critical incident monitoring'. Again, as mentioned in Chapter 4, it is a highly effective method of identifying key areas in practice that may need addressing. It is not a new technique as it was used in the Second World War to de-brief pilots after missions. In essence, individuals identify an event that has not gone well (or, indeed, that *has* gone well) and then review how the event happened and what lessons may be learnt from this. As a result of this process, systems can be changed, educational needs identified and improvement clearly demonstrated. This analysis may be done during surgery meetings and educational needs identified within the team. Many individuals focus on 'near-misses', such as the wrong prescription given to a patient. However, it can be equally rewarding to dissect events that went well and so achieve a real understanding of good processes, as these may be transferable to other situations.

A typical proforma for significant event analysis is shown in Box 6.1.

Box 6.1: Typical proforma for significant event analysis

Describe the event, both positive and not-so-positive elements.

How did it affect ...

    ... you?
    ... the patient?
    ... the practice?

Could it have been avoided?

How do you prevent a recurrence?

What learning needs or developmental needs has this highlighted ...?

    ... for you personally?
    ... for the primary care team?

PACT data analysis

Every quarter doctors are sent detailed information about their prescribing and that of their practices. This is a rich source of information that can be very useful to analyse. It allows doctors to compare their own prescribing with that of their partners, within their health authority and the comparative data of national prescribing. It may be obvious immediately whether they are 'high antibiotic prescribers' or a 'low statin prescribers'. Although the data is presented in its raw numerical form, care is needed to interpret the significance of the numbers.

For example, if doctors are high antibiotic prescribers, does that mean they are prescribing too much? Does it mean they are the only partner in the practice who actually prescribes antibiotics and all the patients come to them? Do they use the prescription as an exit strategy for patients?

Again, if they are low prescribers of statins it may be worth checking whether they are actually complying with the recommendations for the treatment of hypertensive patients, diabetic patients or indeed hyperlipidaemic patients. In essence, review of the PACT data may provide several useful pointers for doctors' further educational development.

When reviewing the PACT data, doctors should ask themselves the following questions.

* How do my costs compare with my partners and nationally?
* In what disease areas am I a high or low prescriber?
* If high, am I overprescribing?
* If low, am I failing to diagnose the condition?
* Have I reviewed the practice or primary care trust drug formulary?
* Am I complying with the drug formulary?
* Is my prescribing in line with recommendations from NICE and national service frameworks?
* What educational needs does this exercise identify?

Referral rates

Again, this is a rich source of information about doctors' knowledge, clinical interests and patient profiles. Looking at the last six months' referrals, for example, can inform doctors of the clinical areas that they refer the most and the least. Just like prescribing details care is needed when interpreting the data. It is well-known that doctors with a special interest in a subject (like clinical assistants) are high referrers in that subject. This clearly does not mean that they are inappropriate referrals but that the individuals have a good understanding of the available appropriate treatment that secondary care can provide. Also, Rowland (1999) stated that only 50% of all referrals are under the direct control of GPs. They may be patient-generated or part of a follow-up programme. More interestingly for individuals is a better understanding of the types of patients they are seeing and needing to refer.

Doctors should ask themselves the following questions.

- Which clinical areas do I refer the most? The least?
- Is it always for the same problem?
- How does this compare with my partners' referral rates?
- Could the condition be treated in the primary care setting? (An example might be referrals for minor surgery.)
- Do I refer because I do not know what to do with the patient or do I refer for a procedure (for example, endoscopy)?
- What educational needs does this identify?

It is also worth checking the replies to referral letters.

- Did you get the diagnosis correct?
- Did you send it to the right department!
- What did you learn about the management of the condition that you did not know before?
- Was it an appropriate referral?
- Could you have done more before the referral was made? (For example, more investigations that could have speeded up the management of the patient.)

This process will identify educational needs and can have a great effect on whether doctors need to refer patients, or what more they can do for them before writing the referral letter.

Investigation rates

A similar thought process is required when looking at the rates of investigations that doctors undertake. Doctors can ask a member of staff to collate the investigations they undertake by checking them against a list of investigations. The member of staff will tick the boxes when the results are returned to the practice. This is a more accurate method than doctors recording the data themselves as not all patients actually show up to have their bloods taken. Doctors may want to gather more information than just the raw numbers of tests. They can also look to see how many tests come back as abnormal compared to the number of normal returns. They can look at the number of tests they order, compared to the number of patients with the disease in the practice. This can be quite revealing.

For example, a local practice which undertook this exercise realised that one of its partners could not possibly be diagnosing thyroid disease as the number of tests per year undertaken by this individual was negligible. Clearly, a learning need had been identified for the individual.

In practice, therefore, it is worth giving a member of staff a list of all the tests undertaken. This should include all blood tests, X-rays, ultrasounds and urine samples. The staff member can then check the returning results and tick the number of tests requested by the doctor and also if the test was normal. Doctors may then ask themselves the following questions.

- Am I a high investigator?
- Do I seem to always send off the same tests?
- What percentage of my tests are abnormal?
- Do I do investigations in each disease category?
- Which conditions do I investigate the least?
- Do I investigate in appropriate numbers for the demography of the practice in terms of mortality and morbidity?
- Do I follow X-ray department guidelines on the investigation of musculoskeletal problems?

It may be important to review the use of investigations as the information gleaned may provide a guide to further educational needs. There can be a tendency to think that GPs overinvestigate because many tests come back normal, but a normal result can be very reassuring for patients. However, there are still areas in which patients are underinvestigated, notably in cholesterol management and the diagnosis of hyperlipidaemia.

Content of national service frameworks

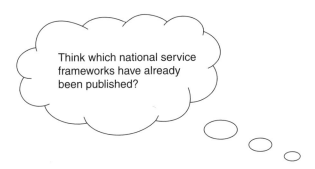

Think which national service frameworks have already been published?

If you do not know you can check the Department of Health (DoH) website (www.doh.gov.uk) or e-mail (dhmail@doh.gsi. gov.uk). Within each of these documents is a list of criteria and targets to be met by primary care teams over the coming years. These can be about audits that have to be undertaken, or increased recording of the particular condition and disease parameters that are applicable in the national service framework, or which partner is the clinical lead in a practice for the national service framework?

The national service frameworks are a rich source of material to look at and see if they highlight educational needs for doctors or their practices. A good example is the criteria in the national service framework for care of the elderly. Within this document practices have to review the medications of all patients every year and every 'six months' for those on five or more items. This is a systems change within practices and doctors will need to know how to implement this change. Again, within this national service framework is the need to develop a disease register for all patients with osteoporosis. Do you know how you would undertake this task?

All the national service frameworks contain tasks that will need to be done by all practices, and will therefore produce task-oriented or problem-oriented strands that may highlight doctors' educational needs.

Local health improvement programmes

Health improvement programmes are being run in each locality.

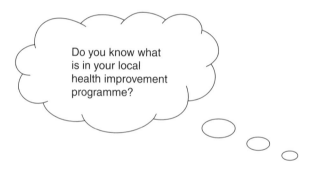

The content of the health improvement programmes in most localities should relate to the specific needs of the local population. This is not an easy thing to define as, although you think that the public health department could give a macro view of health needs, it seldom operates at that level. In reality, many primary care organisations sought to focus health improvement programmes on the national 'must-do' national service frameworks. This has meant that health improvement programmes have invariably been concerned with mental health and cardiovascular disease. In fairness some primary care organisations have been more imaginative and looked at, for example, the needs of the ethnic population within their locality.

By being aware of health improvement programmes and what is actually expected of practices with regard to health improvement, training and educational needs may be highlighted.

Good Medical Practice for General Practitioners

This is, in fact, a document that all GPs received, both in its draft form (RCGP/GPC, 1999) and its final version in March 2002. It is a joint publication from the RCGP and the General Practitioners Committee (GPC). The document sets out to describe what is expected of GPs and why each particular aspect of care is important to them. They are described under seven broad headings.

1   Good clinical care.
2   Maintaining good medical practice.
3   Relationships with patients.
4   Working with colleagues.
5   Teaching and training, assessment and appraisal.
6   Probity.
7   Health and performance of other doctors.

Good Medical Practice for General Practitioners is essential reading for all GPs; it highlights in each section some points that describe an 'excellent GP' and some that describe an 'unacceptable GP'.

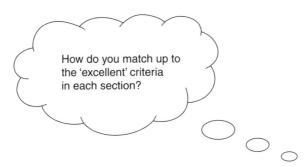
How do you match up to the 'excellent' criteria in each section?

For example, the excellent GP:

• makes sound management decisions, which are based on good practice and evidence.

The unacceptable GP:

• shows little evidence of a coherent or rational approach to diagnosis.

This document forms the backbone of the revalidation process and it is therefore important to have a good grasp of its contents and criteria.

Patient satisfaction surveys

There is increasing emphasis on the need for primary health-care teams to engage the public in meaningful discussion about the services provided and what their actual needs are. A patient survey is a quick and relatively easy method of engaging the patient group. Many practices have active patient participation groups and may feel that they already have a good line of communication with their patients. This may well be the case but even if this is true it is worth looking to a wider cross-section of the patient population to elicit views on the service. One of the problems with asking questions, of any nature, is the potential to raise expectations. If, for example, doctors ask patients if they would like longer appointments with the doctor or in-house physiotherapist, patients may feel that by answering 'yes' that the new service will be provided. Questionnaire design is therefore not easy and doctors should be careful what they include and exclude.

A good example of a patient satisfaction questionnaire is contained in the documentation for the Quality Practice Award from the RCGP. One of the major results of this type of interaction with the patient population is that it will involve doctors in the management of change within their practices. There are unlikely to be clinical areas that are highlighted in a survey so the bulk of the recommendations will be about system changes. Many newly qualified GPs feel that their training has not equipped them with skills in change management so this might well provide the impetus to develop these skills.

Audit

This remains a central tool for individuals and practices when assessing the standards being achieved. Doctors have all under-taken audit as a part of summative assessment and, for most of them, this will have been the eight-point audit completing the full audit cycle.

It is worth using the template of the eight-point criteria when conducting subsequent audits. The criteria are as follows.

1   Reason for choice of audit. (Potential for change/relevant to the practice.)
2   Criterion/criteria chosen. (Relevant to audit subject and justifiable, for example current literature.)
3   Standards set. (Target towards a standard with a suitable timescale.)
4   Preparing and planning. (Evidence of teamwork and adequate discussion, where appropriate.)
5   Data collection (1). (Results compared against standard.)
6   Changes to be evaluated. (Actual example described.)
7   Data collection (2). (Comparison with data collection (1) and standard.)
8   Conclusions (summary of main issues learnt.)

Although it may seem cumbersome to be this formal when doing practice audits, it does make the issues easy to read and understand for all members of the team. Audit allows doctors to implement change and the complete audit cycle allows them to demonstrate improvement. One of the advantages of audits is that they can identify areas for improvement that are transferable elsewhere in the practice. If templates are not being filled in for one of the chronic diseases then it is likely that they are not being filled in for others. The ability to look laterally after an audit can add an extra dimension to the information and learning opportunities made available.

Summary

There are many tools to help individuals to develop their own curriculum.

- It is important to look across the breadth of opportunities in both looking to find gaps in knowledge and performance.
- A good understanding of the preferred method of learning may help doctors better judge the learning opportunities that present themselves.
- The national directives that individuals and practices have to fulfil can provide a rich source of learning opportunities. They can provide good opportunities to improve practice, patient care and the change management skills of individuals.

References

Calman K (1998) *A Review of Continuing Professional Development in General Practice*. DoH, London.

Entwhistle N and Ramsden P (1983) *Understanding Student Learning*. Croom Helm, London.

Eve R (1994) Meeting educational needs in general practice: with PUNs and DENs. *Education for General Practice.*

Eve R (2000) Learning with PUNs and DENs: a method for determining educational needs and the evaluation of its use in primary care. *Education for General Practice* **11**, 73–79.

Honey P and Mumford A (1986) *Using Your Learning Styles.* Peter Honey, Maidenhead.

Honey P and Mumford A (1992) *The Manual of Learning Styles.* Peter Honey, Maidenhead.

Joint Committee for Education (JCE) (1998) *Postgraduate Training for General Practice.* JCE, London.

Perry WG (1981) Cognitive and ethical growth: the making of meaning. In: AW Chickering (ed.) *The Modern American College.* Jossey-Bass, London.

Rowland M (1999) Quality efficiency: enemies or partners. *British Journal of General Practice* **49**, 140–143.

Royal College of General Practitioners (RCGP)/General Practitioners Committee (GPC) (1999) *Good Medical Practice for General Practitioners.* Royal College of General Practitioners, London.

Valley K (1997) Learning styles and courseware design. *Association for Learning Technology Journal* **5**, 42–51.

7

Action learning and learning groups

Introduction

In HPE, as elsewhere in healthcare education, it has become trendy to talk of 'learning sets'. Recently, we have heard colleagues from around the country, who are involved in organising HPE, make statements like these:

'There's a learning set studying for MRCGP'

'We divide them up into locality learning sets'

'Each tutor runs a learning set'

'We try to encourage action learning.'

Are they all talking about the same thing? Is any group of learners a 'learning set'? Does it matter? Why are there whole books (McGill and Beaty, 1992; Revans, 1998; Weinstein, 1998) written about action learning, as well as an 'Institute of Action Learning' (www.action-learning.org) and even a 'University of Action Learning' (www.u-a-l.org)? Are all learning sets involved in action learning? To answer some of these questions, we are going to first look back at the roots of 'action learning' and then address some of the practical issues for HPE.

Defining the terms

Definitions seem like a safe place to start, except that action learning tries hard to be a 'definition-free zone'. Action learners disrespect definitions, as the learning is all about small groups exploring together, groping for shared understanding of problematic concepts. The learning process is almost inseparable from a research process, as new knowledge and understanding is being created and shared.

Example: definitions rejected

The worked examples are based on a fictitious group of six HPE learners from different parts of the same county, who decided to get together to work on 'The Difficult Consultation'. They are referred to as the 'consultations learning set'.

> At its first meeting, the group did not waste much time defining 'The Difficult Consultation,' as this would not be of much practical help. Rather, it was decided that each of the learners would introduce cases they had encountered and which seemed difficult, for whatever reason, and the group would discuss the cases together. The objective was to gradually evolve a common understanding of what makes consulting difficult under what circumstances.

There are a number of concepts that overlap, and perhaps the most helpful way of illustrating the extent of the territory is to list some relevant keywords.

Keywords associated with action learning

- learning sets
- reflection (on action and in-action)
- insightful questioning
- action research
- collaborative enquiry
- small group facilitation

Action learning

The founder of action learning was Reg Revans, a Cambridge physicist in the 1930s, who realised the importance of empowering learners, rather than glorifying teachers (Levy and Delahoussaye, 2000). Revans (1980) realised that if we can concentrate on what we *do not* know, rather than on what we do know, we can promote a process of questioning and reflection which can be highly productive for learning. He is known for the equation

$$L = P + Q$$

where L (learning) occurs through P (programmed knowledge) in conjunction with Q (insightful questioning).

Example: Revans' formula

The 'consultations learning set' analysed what it had learnt after a few sessions. All those in the set found that they had picked up new approaches to difficult consultations (L). They had done this by teasing out the difficult aspects of each case they had discussed (Q) and relating this to what they knew of the theory of consulting in general practice, drawing on models such as 'Pendleton', 'Neighbour', 'Cambridge Calgary' (P). Both P and Q were essential components of L.

Learning sets

Integral to this notion of learning through uncertainty was the experience of learning with others, in what have now become 'action learning sets' (Table 7.1). Revans, who had benefited enormously from the learning community at the Rutherford Physics

Laboratory, talked about a tight learning community where 'real people are obliged to tackle real problems in real time'.

Table 7.1:   Learning sets*

Attributes of a learning set (after Revans)	HPE example
Small stable group ('set') of about six 'comrades in adversity' working in a regular social process	HPE learning sets sometimes formed during the vocational training scheme year, or sometimes have a situation in common (for example, non-principals)
Activities lead to examination of the problem(s) and the self	Personal and professional development issues for the doctor are always considered
Target the reality of the 'mess' at field level	Not afraid to tackle the realities of working in today's NHS
Problems are complex and have no identifiable solution	For example, achieving a sustainable home/work balance; maximising accessibility to patients
Issues have significance and risk for the participants	For example, group exploring patient complaints
Process issues	May be self-facilitating, or facilitated by HPE tutor
The group proceeds by conjecture and refutation	
Exchanges advice, criticism and support	
Learning is both defined and accidental	
Learn from and with each other to take observable action	

*Adapted from International Foundation for Action Learning.

Action research

At around the same time that Revans was promulgating action learning, others were developing the principles of action research, following the work of Lewin (1946), an American social researcher and passionate community worker of the immediate post-war period. Lewin emphasised the need for joint studies of social scientists and practitioners and the elements of action research were laid out as a four-stage cycle of planning, acting, observing and reflecting.

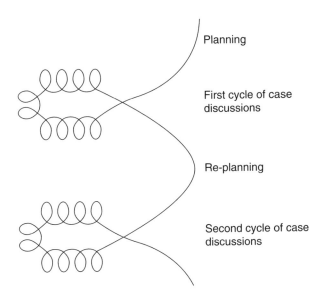

Figure 7.1: An example of action research spirals in a learning set (Peile, 2000a).

In this example of a multidisciplinary learning set, working with case discussions, each case discussion, represented as a small spiral loop, followed loosely Lewin's (1946) cycle.

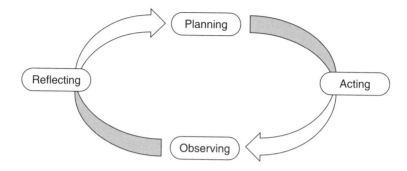

Figure 7.2: Lewin's (1946) four-stage cycle of planning, acting, observing and reflecting.

Each *series* of case discussions formed a cycle in a bigger spiral. The parallels with action learning do not end there. The following descriptions are from experts in the field.

- Action research aims to contribute both to the practical concerns of people in an immediate problematic situation and to the goals of social science by joint collaboration within a mutually acceptable ethical framework.

    (Rapoport, 1970)

- Action research seeks to decentralise traditional research by maintaining a commitment to local contexts rather than to the quest for truth and to liberate research from its excessive reliance on the restrictive conventional rules of the research game.

    (Marshall and Rossman, 1999)

- Action research is a form of self-reflexive enquiry undertaken by participants in social situations in order to improve the rationality and justice of their own practices, their understanding of these practices and the situations in which these practices are carried out.

    (Carr and Kemmis, 1986)

Note the emphasis on shared concerns, practice-based collaboration, local contexts, reflection and democracy.

Example: from action learning to action research

The 'consultations learning set' was working well. Together its members had grappled with some of the aspects that made consulting difficult, but they found that they had moved past the stage where they were deriving help from published literature on the consultation. Enthused by some of their discussions, they decided to explore further the notion of involving patients more in untangling difficult consultations. They resolved that the next time each of them encountered a consultation which felt difficult, the doctor would ask the patient to reflect on whether it had been difficult for them, and what had made it difficult. At the next meeting, members brought back their experience of this experiment, and together they refined the technique, modifying how they involved the patient in the process. They then faced the decision as to whether to write up their experiences for publication, or whether to be content that between them they had evolved something that was of use in their everyday practice.

Activity theory

Before we move on from the world of the theorists to the practical considerations for action learning in HPE, there is this one last topic to mention.

You may have noticed a political element creeping into definitions of action research. Activity theory is even more political, having reference to themes which start with Engels and Marx. The great modern exponent of activity theory is Yrgo Engestrom who stated:

'Development can be understood by tracing disruptions, troubles, and innovations at the level of concrete modes of the activity, both historical and current. The analysis of such data leads to hypothetical identification of the internal contradictions of the activity system.' (Engestrom, 1993, p. 72)

Complex it certainly is, but Engestrom's concept is not that different from that of Neighbour, who encourages us to look for the turbulence in a consultation (Neighbour, 1987).

Example: looking for turbulence in the consultation

Here is one of the cases which an HPE learner brought to the learning set.

> Mrs X was a frequent consulter. Very overweight and always polite and considerate of her doctor, she usually had a smiling face, which was somewhat at odds with the tales of woe, which came tumbling out in different consultations. I had yet to fathom out what 'made her tick'. I wanted to practise the micro-skills outlined in Neighbour's (1987) 'inner consultation' and I found myself listening intently not so much to *what* she was saying but to *how* she was saying it. I risked a probe, 'Do you know, Mary, twice today, your voice has slowed down, your smile has become a bit strained, and you have had a sort of nervous giggle: both times have been when you have been talking about your mother. Do you want to tell me a bit about her?' We struck gold, and consultations have never been the same since. Once we were able to talk about a really important pain in her life, and look at how to make it bearable, Mary was able to deal with numerous other discomforts without any help from me.

Activity theory is all about understanding by looking at patterns and concentrating on the disruptions in those patterns to further our understanding of something problematic. Engestrom believes that textbook theory is of limited value: activity theorists hold that you can only study meaningful theory in the *workplace context*. Note the connection here around *action* and *activity*. Action learning, action research and activity theory are all about 'on-the-job' learning, reflecting and changing. Hence the relevance to HPE, which is designed to get practitioners learning in, and about, the workplace and, through their learning, changing what goes on in the workplace.

A good example of 'work as a testbench of theory' came in Engestrom's (1993) analysis of a Finnish primary care system, and he demonstrates beautifully the benefits to healthcare of looking at where the system is not working smoothly.

Example of activity theory

Engestrom and colleagues were commissioned to look at the reorganisation of primary medical care in Espoo, Finland, and they started by analysing some doctor–patient consultations by use of an interpersonal recall technique (Engestrom, 1993). Engestrom makes a valuable contribution to the methodology of consultation analysis with his tools for looking at dysfunction by means of identifying discoordinations by categorising the qualities of the doctor–patient relationship, by use of perspectives gleaned from the consultation. Activity theory is complex, but for those who are interested, Chaiklin and Lave (1993) offer numerous case examples from different fields. The relevance to HPE is probably for those high-flyers who are interested in looking at the world of general practice more widely – perhaps to make changes across primary care trusts. For such movers and shakers, activity theory is a powerful tool because it grounds theory in practice; the context is very clearly that of the real workplace of today, examined in an historical perspective so that change may be proposed which is likely to work, because it takes account of where all the stakeholders are coming from, what are their drivers and how they interact.

Transcript from stimulated recall interviews:

> Engestrom looks at what is going on in the consultation in terms of an historical framework of doctor–patient activity. In other

words: 'Where is the patient coming from? Where is the doctor coming from?' He attempts to examine where the craftwork of general practice fits into the framework, and concludes that there is, as yet, little 'collectively and expansively mastered activity'.

What Engestrom means by this is general practice activity which is working along agreed lines towards agreed ends, and (thinking particularly about activity in the consultation) that GPs should be trained to a level of mastery, which consistently achieves the desired result for patients.

Relevance of action learning, learning sets and action research to HPE

The picture that is emerging of this sort of learning is one that seems to have immediate relevance to young professionals, such as HPE learners:

* learning that involves collaboration with others in committed groups
* learning that values uncertainty
* learning that happens repeatedly over a period of time
* learning that promotes reflection, enquiry and change
* learning that is democratic and takes account of social values
* learning that invokes commitment from learners
* learning that has a research focus: wanting to discover better ways of practice.

Learning how to learn

You may have noticed that a recurring theme throughout this book is 'change management'. Part of the task of HPE seems to be to enable young doctors to cope with the demands of managing change in the NHS. How are we going to learn our new ways of working? It seems that new ways of learning are needed, and there may be something about the 'newness' which helps. This has certainly been the experience over the introduction of intermediate care in our locality (Peile, 2000a).

The worked examples now change to ones based on the real 'new ways of working: new ways of learning' set. This multi-disciplinary group actually met to learn from case discussions about clients they had looked after in the early days of inter-mediate care projects.

Example: true interprofessional learning

Often the case discussions about dependent elderly people, who had required the services of the intermediate care team, included aspects of diabetes management. There was a case about an elderly lady who had brittle diabetes. The support worker who had been caring for her learnt from the district nurse the import-ance of insulin timings, relative to food. The district nurse learnt something she did not know about the importance of complex carbohydrates in smoothing blood sugar oscillations. In this instance it was the doctor who filled in the gap in her know-ledge, but the learning was reciprocated as the GP was pleased to learn about the practicalities of leaving insulin drawn up in the fridge. The key to sorting out the problem of hypos was, however, held by the support worker, who asked, 'Do you think it matters that she never eats until the dog has been fed, and if she can't find the dog, there may be a long time between getting her insulin and having her dinner?' In this case the contextual know-ledge was every bit as valuable as the theoretical knowledge. The GP left this case discussion determined to think more about 'life as it is lived', and not just to consider the causes of insulin resistance!

The Centre for the Advancement of Interprofessional Learning (CAIPE) definition of interprofessional learning involves profes-sionals of different disciplines learning *'with, from* and *about* each other, *to facilitate collaboration in practice'** (Barr, 1998). It can be very rewarding to bring learners together, who have a common purpose, and then to get them to think about the process of their learning.

*Note that interprofessional learning is a subset of multidisciplinary learning, where workers of different disciplines learn together for whatever purpose.

We talk elsewhere (*see* Chapter 6) about learning styles. Learners who are going to work together in groups may find it helpful to know something of their own and each others' learning styles. It can help to understand and facilitate the group process, moving the group safely into new ways of learning.

Checks and balances for action learning in HPE

Action learning is no different from other forms of learning. It needs a certain amount of enthusiasm, rigour and intellectual honesty if it is to be productive. Above all, it needs to be fun and stimulating. One danger for learning sets is that they can degenerate into cosy chat sessions, where people just swap anecdotes or have a general and purposeless moan about the current state of general practice! Think back to Revans' (1980) equation:

$$L = P + Q$$

Learning will not occur without programmed knowledge in conjunction with insightful questioning.

Here are a few questions that a learning set may want to ask itself in the early days.

- Is this the right grouping for this learning purpose?
- Do we have a common interest in learning about the areas we are discussing?
- Is the group diverse enough in its thinking or experience to challenge our thinking, or do we need to invite others with a different perspective or professional background?

It is a hallmark of functional learning sets that they value diversity.

And then there are some questions that help an established learning set to audit itself.

- Are we highlighting the areas of knowledge, skills and attitudes which we need to develop, and do we help each

other think about how to go about developing ourselves
further?

- How do we incorporate evidence-based practice in our
  learning?
- Where there does not seem to be evidence out there to help
  us, can we construct the evidence to help others? (See example
  below.)
- Are we keeping our discussions focused on 'real-life general
  practice'?
- Are we thinking broadly enough? Do we need to think more
  laterally to find examples from other worlds, which bear on
  the problems we are discussing?

Example: finding evidence to help when there seems to be no evidence

The 'new ways of working: new ways of learning' set was
considering the case of an elderly, rather depressed lady. The
support worker, who had opened up a can of worms of unresolved
grief by asking the old lady if she wanted to talk about her son's
death, asked the group, 'I've not been trained as a counsellor;
should I have done that? Could I have done more harm than
good?' Her question was eventually formulated in evidence-
based terms as: 'Does an opportunity to talk about unresolved
loss to an empathic caregiver (untrained in counselling) change
health or psychological well-being in older depressed patients?'
Databases were searched (MEDLINE, Embase, PsycLIT, CINAHL
and Sociofile) for the following search terms: *reminiscence, life-
review, communication, listening, empathy, depression, counselling,
psychotherapy, social support, caregiving, confidant* and *bereave-
ment*. All shed some light on the question but none directly, so
a novel approach was adopted of deriving evidence by a series
of assertion steps, and this was eventually published (Peile,
2000b) (*see* Figure 7.3).

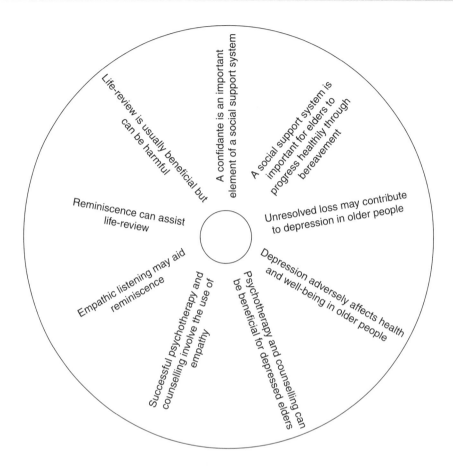

Figure 7.3: Deriving evidence by a series of assertion steps (Peile, 2000b).

What are the blocks to action learning?

It really is quite amazing. Get willing learners together in small groups and learning happens, in HPE as in other situations. Usually – but not always. What goes wrong? Sometimes the problem is lack of common purpose, and here the checklist of questions for a group to ask itself may come in very useful.

Think back to learning needs assessment (Chapter 4). If the topics that the group is addressing are not on the learners' agenda, it is unlikely that learners are going to engage fully in the learning set. HPE learners have had recent experience of working in groups on the day release of the vocational training scheme, looking at topics which are often suggested by course organisers to fit in with the training curriculum. Some will have had bad experiences of these 'one-size-fits-all' learning groups. HPE is time for something different. Across the country there have been many early experiments in delivering HPE, and as yet little evidence has emerged as to 'best practice'. The best learning sets are those where the group comes together voluntarily with a common learning purpose.

This is not to argue for homogeneity in learning sets. It has already been stated that one hallmark of a good group is that it values diversity. There is much to be gained from multidisciplinary learning sets where interprofessional learning is likely to occur (remember the definition of interprofessional learning: 'learning *with, from* and *about* each other, to *facilitate collaboration in practice*'). Conversely, tokenism in multidisciplinary learning is actually counterproductive: working together can be damaged by attempting learning experiences where someone of one discipline is alienated by lack of relevant experience or by lack of familiarity with the language or approaches used by others. Like working together, the benefits of learning together need to be debated, rather than just accepted as fashionable (Campbell and Johnson, 1999). For as Leathard (1994) points out, there is at least a possibility that studying in multiprofessional groups can 'erode professional values or, worse, entrench negative stereotypes that professions hold about one another'.

Checklist for multidisciplinary learning sets

- Has each member relevant experience to contribute on an equal footing?
- Does each member share the common learning objectives, even if approaching from a different angle?
- Can the group talk a common language, accessible to all?
- Is the group prepared to be even-handed in valuing the diversity of different approaches to a problem, based on different professional backgrounds?
- Can each member contribute to the learning of others and are they all prepared to learn from the others?

What makes a good group?

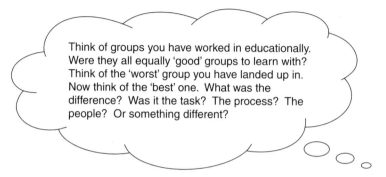

Think of groups you have worked in educationally. Were they all equally 'good' groups to learn with? Think of the 'worst' group you have landed up in. Now think of the 'best' one. What was the difference? Was it the task? The process? The people? Or something different?

Does your list look something like the one shown in Table 7.2?

Table 7.2: What makes a good group

Features of 'good' groups	Features of 'bad' groups
Common purpose	All after different things
Explicit ground rules	No boundaries to group discussion – people quite disrespectful of each other
Valuing diversity	Intolerant of difference
All members contributing	Group space hogged by some whilst others stay quite quiet and peripheral
Able to balance 'task' and 'process'	So task-oriented that nobody gives any thought to group process, and learning gets ignored, or else endlessly navel-gazing to the point where the group frustrates its members by achieving little
Fun – space for harmless laughter and enjoyment	Uncomfortable, even threatening or unsafe for some group members

Much has been written about functional and dysfunctional groups and we would suggest that all who engage in a learning set should give some thought to the process, perhaps reading one of the many good books on the subject (for example Elwyn *et al.*, 2000).

Facilitation issues?

If so much hinges on the functionality of a learning set, should the group be facilitated, say, by an HPE tutor? There is no one answer to this question, as undoubtedly some learning sets function very well on self-facilitation. The role of the HPE tutor here may just be to make life easy in terms of supporting a convenient place to meet and perhaps prompting the group to think about its ground rules and not to neglect process issues.

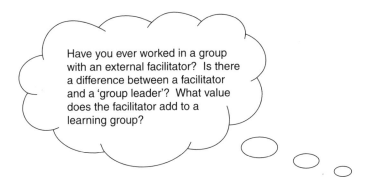

Have you ever worked in a group with an external facilitator? Is there a difference between a facilitator and a 'group leader'? What value does the facilitator add to a learning group?

There is a lot to be said for skilled facilitation in some situations, and sometimes this function may just be a temporary one; the facilitator can be there as the group 'forms' and 'storms' and then leave it to its own devices as it 'norms' (Tuckman, 1965). (For a good explanation of the Tuckman stages in the life of small groups and for some thoughts and checklists about group leadership styles *see* www.nwlink.com/~donclark/leader/leadtem2.html.)

Ongoing work on facilitation has included looking at some 20 transcripts of the 'new ways of working: new ways of learning' set. Case history discussions are an effective form of multidisciplinary team learning, focusing discussion on the common concern – patients (Peile, 2000a). In this way, existing perspectives can broaden to reveal new ways of working as other disciplines contribute to understanding.

There appeared to be a definite role for facilitators here, as the uneven power base of support workers and trained professionals (social workers, therapists, district nurses, GPs, etc.), and their vastly different levels of training and experience, meant that the support workers had to be empowered to speak up and contribute (Peile, 2000a).

By means of coloured highlighting on the transcripts it was possible to conduct an informal discourse analysis, looking at what sort of learning happened under what conditions (Peile and Briner, 2001).

Example: lessons of facilitating an interprofessional learning set

- Technical jargon disempowered and excluded some people, and it is worth agreeing to exclude jargon in the ground rules of the learning set.
- This is only effective if facilitators (or the group members themselves) police the rule gently but effectively: 'Could you rephrase that, because you used technical terms?' Very soon members stop using jargon.
- Shared learning is more likely to happen when learners talk a shared language.
- The initial language sets the tone for later interchanges. In the group the facilitator learnt to invite the support worker to speak first. The tone of the discussion was set by somebody talking in 'homely' language about the patient's life, and everybody could participate. If, on the other hand, the doctor opened the discussion, focusing on technical aspects

of the treatment plan, 'technospeak' became the order of the day and the focus of the learning, narrowing its value.

- Emotional learning needs optimal conditions. When the homely discussions got going, people started to work on important problems dealing with the way we relate to each other and to patients under difficult circumstances. The sharing of feelings was a vital part of the learning for all, but this needed security and confidence to be built up within the group.

Summary

- Action learning and related activities have a lot to offer HPE learners.
- Activity theory is all about connecting learning to the workplace.
- Action learning involves both reflection and a commitment to change.
- Learning sets can be an extraordinarily powerful tool for HPE.
- Effective learning sets need a sense of common purpose among group members.
- Groups of different disciplines do not necessarily learn well together.
- True interprofessional learning happens when professionals learn with, from and about each other in order to facilitate collaboration.
- Attention must be paid to process issues, such as ground rules and facilitation.

References

Barr H (1998) Cochrane review of outcomes from IPE – a work in progress. *CAIPE Bulletin* **15**, 3.

Campbell J and Johnson C (1999) Trend spotting: fashions in medical education. *British Medical Journal* **318**, 1272–1275.

Carr W and Kemmis S (1986) *Becoming Critical: education, knowledge and action research*. Falmer Press, London.

Chaiklin S and Lave J (eds) (1993) *Understanding Practice: perspectives on activity and context*. Cambridge University Press, Cambridge.

Elwyn G, Greenhalgh T *et al.* (2000) *Groups*. Radcliffe Medical Press, Oxford.

Engestrom Y (1993) Developmental studies of work as a testbench of activity theory: the case of primary medical practice. In: S Chaiklin and J Lave (eds) *Understanding Practice: perspectives on activity and context*. Cambridge University Press, Cambridge.

Leathard A (1994) *Inter-professional developments in Britain: an overview. Going Inter-professional*. Routledge, London.

Levy M and Delahoussaye M (2000) Reg Revans: a man of action. *Training Journal*. www.trainingjournal.co.uk

Lewin K (1946) Action research and minority problems. *Journal of Social Issues* **2**, 34–36.

Marshall C and Rossman G (1999) *Designing Qualitative Research*. Sage, Thousand Oaks, CA.

McGill I and Beaty L (1992) *Action Learning*. Kogan Page, London.

Neighbour R (1987) *The Inner Consultation*. MTP Press, London.

Peile E (2000a) *New Ways of Working: New Ways of Learning: action research in the Weston project*. School of Education, Oxford Brookes University.

Peile E (2000b) Is there an evidence base for intuition and empathy? The risks and benefits of inviting an older person to discuss unresolved loss. *Journal of Primary Care Research and Development* **1**, 73–79.

Peile E and Briner W (2001) Team and organisational learning in a cross-functional community of practice: the importance of privileging voices. *Career Development International* **6**, 396–402.

Rapoport R (1970) Three dilemmas of action research. *Human Relations* **23**, 499–513.

Revans R (1980) *Action Learning.* Blond & Briggs, London.

Revans R (1998) *ABC of Action Learning.* Lemos and Crane, London.

Tuckman BW (1965) Developmental sequence in small groups. *Psychological Bulletin* **63**, 384–399.

Weinstein K (1998) *Action Learning.* Gower, London.

8

Planning and delivering education and learning

Innovations

In previous chapters we have discussed what HPE learners think they need to learn. We have also looked at different learning styles, for example activist, reflector, theorist and pragmatist. This chapter examines some of the developments in the process of planning and delivering educational events. Though many of these have a proven track record of facilitating successful learning, the methods of delivery develop continuously as new opportunities present themselves, for example e-learning.

The learning environment

It is important to consider the learning climate, that is, the environment in which learning occurs. If this climate is inappropriate it will undoubtedly influence the learning process, no matter how innovative or sound the method of delivery. How many of us as younger students remember being told by well-meaning parents that 'We couldn't possibly study with that racket going on.' That racket referring to our particular choice in loud pop music. As a more mature learner, would you now echo the sentiment?

Each individual will have their own preferred learning environment (which may included background music varying from The Beatles to baroque) but if you are responsible for delivering learning there are several general conditions to consider. These apply to any learning event and not just HPE.

Noise

Unsolicited noise can be a major distraction and that includes the catering staff setting up teacups and saucers in the same room as the learning event 15 minutes before the session ends.

Space

Size does make a difference. A large area with too few people can feel as uncomfortable as a small area with too many people. Layout is also important; 'theatre' style may be an excellent choice for a lecture or seminar but cabaret style (several small tables) can be a more efficient use of space for small group work.

Climate

It is impossible to suit everyone, but the option to make the environment cooler or warmer is necessary. Do not underestimate the usefulness of a 'fresh air' break to revive concentration.

Timing

Because time is at a premium it is often tempting to cram too much into a learning session. This highlights the importance of curriculum planning, as discussed earlier (p. 103). Any educational event should be properly planned and structured with clear aims and objectives for learning outcome.

Learners may not always be able to control their learning environment. However, developing an understanding of individual preferred options can help them to appreciate why some learning experiences have been more or less effective than others.

Educators will not always be able to provide the optimum learning environment. However, being aware of the problems that learners might experience in the environment should help to minimise the difficulties. They should be prepared to be flexible in their delivery if the unexpected, such as considerable building work outside the 'classroom' window, is encountered.

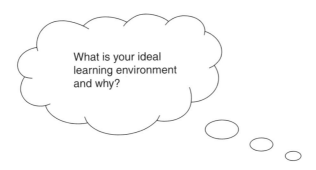

How learning is delivered

Consideration of the ideal learning environment is likely for purely practical reasons to be secondary to consideration about how learning events will be delivered. This may depend on what educators are trying to deliver and whom is being targeted. The following methods will be particularly appropriate for HPE learners and their colleagues from other health professions and disciplines.

Multidisciplinary learning

'All staff should work effectively in teams, appreciating the roles of other staff and agencies involved in the care of patients' (DoH, 2001). Multidisciplinary learning does not mean all members of all disciplines learning the same thing at the same time (Chambers *et al.*, 2002). Multidisciplinary learning has more to do with individuals recognising their role, and the role of others, and learning together in a way that best addresses their needs and meets the needs of the organisation to improve patient care.

'All health professionals should expect their education and training to include common learning with other professionals' (DoH, 2001). Multidisciplinary learning also emphasises that common learning should run from undergraduate and pre-registration programmes through to continuing professional education. In a multidisplinary forum different professionals will, for whatever reason, learn side by side. A subset of multi-disciplinary education is interprofessional education. This is when two professionals learn with, from and about each other to facilitate collaboration in practice (Barr, 2001).

Many members of practice teams will have identified similar learning needs to those of HPE learners. Many of these needs can be satisfied in a multidisciplinary environment, although there will be occasions when uniprofessional learning is appropriate. Multidisciplinary learning is essential for the development of individuals and organisations (Senge, 1990). Multidiscip-linary learning can be a particularly effective and appropriate way of addressing 'core' learning needs, such as management skills, communication and IT skills. It is also an effective way of addressing a team approach to clinical issues (Burton, 2000). However, it is important to recognise that different team members will have different levels of expertise. Failure to take account of this may leave some learners feeling uncomfortable and unconvinced of the value of multidisciplinary learning.

Problem-based learning

Problem-based learning is not a new concept. It was first advocated by Dr Maria Montessori at the beginning of the twentieth century. However, it was not until the 1960s and 1970s that problem-based learning was acknowledged as a beneficial tool in medical education when it was introduced by Howard Burrows (Davis and Harden, 1998). Problem-based learning lends itself effectively to both unidisciplinary and multidisciplinary learning.

What is problem-based learning?

Boud (1985) suggests that the starting point for problem-based learning is a problem, which learners wish to solve. The learning experience is not simply about problem-solving, although this may be part of the process. Ross (1991) suggests that learners 'must identify and search for the knowledge they need to obtain in order to approach the problem'.

The role of the problem is not necessarily to be solved but to act as a stimulus for learning. The problem scenario can cover a range of issues, for example clinical, ethical or management. However, when designing a problem scenario educators must be clear about the learning objectives and ensure that the problem will enable students to learn the appropriate material to meet the objectives. 'Learning should be organised around problems which are related to the profession rather than around the academic subjects' (Boud, 1985).

How does problem-based learning work?

To be conducted effectively problem-based learning (like all learning) needs an appropriate amount of protected time. Downey and O'Brien (2001) suggest between one and a half and two hours as ideal. The size of the group is likely to be between six and ten people, which may mean subdividing larger groups if necessary. Groups will need facilitators with good small group facilitation skills. Additionally, facilitators must understand the process of problem-based learning. Davis and Harden (1998) suggest that the difference between small group facilitators and problem-based learning facilitators is that problem-based learning facilitators must not provide information but allow learners to seek out the information for themselves.

The stages of problem-based learning

* The group is given the problem scenario in a written format.
* This may need to be distributed individually or the group may nominate a reader.
* The group may also nominate an individual to keep brief notes.
* Through discussion the group identifies the learning issues (initially this stage may be done independently with the group reconvening to discuss individual and group learning objectives).
* Having identified the learning issues the group will decide which ones they are going to address and how this will be done.
* The group will have an action plan of what is needed to address the learning issues. This may include information or data-gathering, literature searches or discussions with other health professionals and team members.
* The group will then reconvene after an appropriate time (possibly two to three weeks) to discuss the knowledge acquired. This may, in turn, raise more learning issues.

Problem-based learning is a useful and effective way of encouraging team learning. It enables the subject matter to be learnt in context. It is an active type of learning and allows learners (HPE or otherwise) to take more responsibility for their learning.

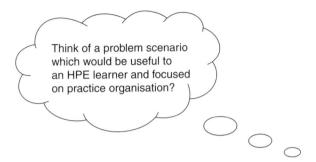

Think of a problem scenario which would be useful to an HPE learner and focused on practice organisation?

Jigsaw learning

Another form of problem-based learning is 'jigsaw learning'. With this method, several learners work independently on one part of a learning task. It is important to ensure that all parts of the learning task are covered. Learners working on the same part of the learning task then come together to compare and discuss their responses and check their understanding against that of other learners. Learners then reform into groups in which each of the different parts of the task is represented. Individual learners then explain to the others their response to their part of the problem (Aronson *et al.*, 1978).

Mentoring

'Mentoring is the process of helping another learn and enhance their professional role' (Watkins and Whalley, 1993).

The role of the mentor can be wide-ranging. Morton-Cooper and Palmer (1993) suggest that at different times mentors may be called upon to be any one of the following:

- adviser
- counsellor
- role-model
- facilitator

- coach
- networker
- teacher.

The role may evolve as the relationship of mentor and mentee matures, and the needs of the mentee or the reason for creating the mentorship change and develop. Doctors completing their vocational training scheme will have had a trainer who has acted as educational supervisor and who may then be asked to make the transition to mentor. If this is the case, the trainer and the newly qualified GP must be quite clear about the different roles. As an educational supervisor, the trainer has a responsibility towards the learner for monitoring outcome. However, this is certainly not the case in the role of mentor.

Mentoring is a developing area in the general practice setting. Although some doctors and team members have embraced the concept, this has been done on an informal basis. The pace of change within the NHS during the last few years has highlighted the need for a more formal supportive framework (Freeman, 1998). Though this is still yet to happen, government initiatives such as GP appraisal will help to focus on mentoring as a learning tool. This is a particularly supportive mechanism for HPE learners, who may feel isolated as they make the transition from registrar to GP.

A Standing Committee on Postgraduate Medical and Dental Education (SCOPME) (1998) report on mentoring listed the following factors as contributing to the need for support for doctors:

- changing roles in the last ten years
- increasing workloads
- lack of opportunities for informal peer support
- need for educational support
- increasing concern about the retention of doctors in some specialities.

Four years on the issues remain the same.

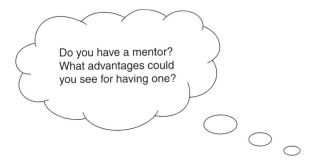

Do you have a mentor?
What advantages could
you see for having one?

The qualities of a mentor

There is no definitive list. The following is an amalgam of suggestions from several sources (Carruthers, 1993; Brockbank, 1994; Freeman, 1998; Connor *et al.*, 2000):

- team player
- active listener
- has the respect of peers
- flexible in their thinking
- non-judgemental
- self-confident
- good communicator
- knowledgeable
- committed to mentoring
- observes confidentiality
- networker
- open-minded.

Freeman (1998) goes on to suggest that undesirable attributes include:

- concrete thinking
- power-seeking
- controlling
- poor communication skills.

Both the mentor and the mentee roles should be voluntary, and there must be mutual respect between the two individuals. Mentor and mentee should feel at ease in each other's company. The frequency of the meetings should be mutually agreed. The intervals between meetings should be relevant to the situation. It is important that they do not simply become a habit and therefore reduce the possible benefits of the process. Contact does not always have to be face-to-face, but remember that body language is lost in most electronic communications.

Although mentoring may be used to support individuals through personal and professional issues it is also a useful educational tool. Mentors can assist their mentees in unravelling the complexities of their learning needs and discuss how they would feel most comfortable about addressing these needs. Mentors may be able to direct mentees towards available resources but must take care not to tell them what to do. It is not the role of a mentor to act as disciplinarian for unfinished tasks. When mentoring is used as an educational tool it is essential that the education agenda is that of the mentee and not that of the mentor (Freeman, 1998).

e-learning

The widespread availability and accessibility of computer hardware and software programmes has allowed us not only to communicate electronically but also to learn electronically. However, the underlying principles of learning must not be ignored when promoting e-learning. e-learning should complement other methods of learning. It should not be considered as a panacea for the delivery of inexpensive learning to as many learners as possible. Educators must be able to evaluate the quality of the learning programme. If educators plan to design their own programmes they must avoid certain pitfalls. It is worth remembering that when we communicate, either to an individual or make a presentation to a group:

- 55% of the information we receive from other people is given in the body language, including eye contact
- 38% from the intonation of what they say
- 7% from the actual words they use (Mehrabian and Ferris, 1967).

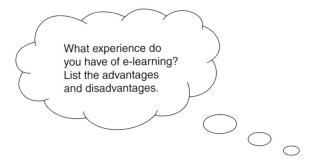

What experience do you have of e-learning? List the advantages and disadvantages.

The e-learning programme

The same principles apply whether you are evaluating a commercial package or whether you are designing your own package.

Support

We do not learn effectively in isolation and the drop-out rate among e-learners is 50% – considerably higher than among those learning by more traditional methods, such as distance learning (20%) and classroom-based learning (7%) (Wilkinson, 2000). e-learners need to feel part of their learning community and should be able to communicate with other learners undertaking the same programme. This can be done through 'chat rooms' or 'online' discussion groups, but learners must receive an explicit invitation to contribute to the discussion. A similar mechanism should be set up to allow easy communication with the tutor or course organiser.

Ease of use

If a programme is too complicated to use it is unlikely to facilitate successful learning. It must be clear from the outset what prior knowledge is required by learners to enable them to work through the programme. If there is no prerequisite knowledge then learners should be reassured of this to maintain their confidence levels. Instructions should be clear and talk directly to learners. An effective programme will have a menu or an index that allows learners to navigate their way around the system. It should also allow them to move backwards through the programme in order to check out and consolidate what they have already encountered. The use of colour graphics and pictures can make the programme more inviting, but these should be relevant and not gratuitous.

Content

There is sometimes a tendency to use material as e-learning that is still better suited to printed material. A programme that consists of many pages of text to be read by learners or even to be printed out by them is likely to be more effective left in book form. What you may have here is a useful resource rather than a learning course! It is also worth remembering that whereas we recognise that a book will date, our expectation of electronic products is that they will be updated continually. Some programmes will appear at first sight to be very good because of their presentation and interactive style. However, they may be light on relevant content and not deliver the anticipated learning opportunities. Not all e-learning will necessarily be done sitting at the computer. The programme may direct or suggest to learners that they do something practical, such as making a model or interviewing a colleague. Some e-learning programmes will have sound as well as text. These may show individuals talking through the programme. Whilst this may seem enticing educators should be aware of the danger of 'passive' learning.

A lecture is a lecture even if the delivery appears to be smart and trendy.

An effective e-learning package will have:

- clearly defined learning outcomes and objectives
- clear and direct instructions
- the facility for learners to communicate with other learners and the course organiser
- easy navigation
- stated clearly the required prior level of knowledge
- content appropriate to e-learning
- been interactive and attractive to use.

If educators are designing their own packages it is absolutely essential that they are piloted. If possible, programmes should be tested on someone with the lowest level of competence required to use them. Consider the learning styles we have talked about in Chapter 6 and try to include something for everyone. Tell learners at the outset how long the programme should take so they know if they have sufficient time. Lastly, if humour is used (and it can be effective) test it out on several people to ensure that the programme is really saying what you think it is. Remember, words without body language and intonation often lose something in interpretation.

Distance learning

e-learning can lend itself to distance learning. Distance learning is an increasingly popular way for individuals to undertake certificates, diplomas, degrees and higher degrees. The advantage of distance learning is its flexibility – learners determine when and where they study and how much or how little they study. Distance learning packages are also usually comparatively low in cost.

However, there are also disadvantages and it is important for all learners, including our HPE cohorts, to be realistic about the demands distance learning can make. Hartley *et al.* (2001) suggest that (as with e-learning) working in isolation does not allow students to talk to each other and to share learning experiences. These authors stress the importance of developing support networks, both with other learners and with tutors, lecturers and administrators. Many distance learning packages offer an opportunity for short residential or summer school study. This peer group support is as important as the learning material. The duration of a distance learning course can be lengthy (several years in fact). Learners are unlikely to work as fast as they think they will and maintaining motivation can be difficult. They must also allow for 'life events'. Over a three to four year period things will inevitably happen that affect either learners' ability or capacity to study as much as they hoped they would. Some distance learning courses progress through certificate, diploma and masters stages and allow learners to defer at a 'convenient' stopping place but still achieve a level of accredited learning.

Distance learning can be a very positive experience, with a rewarding sense of achievement. It does require commitment and a level of personal organisation to ensure that learners balance their studies with their professional and family lives. They should remember the importance of networking with other students and also share their experiences, positive and negative, with family and colleagues. Their support is invaluable particularly when the going feels tough!

Concept mapping

This is a visual representation of meaningful relationships between concepts in the form of propositions. It allows learners to visually represent connections and relationships between concepts, ideas and information. Candy (1991) suggests that this allows students to externalise their understanding. It also allows them to put it into a format that may be read and interpreted by others. This format might be used by HPE learners when discussing organisational issues within the NHS.

Experiential learning

This approach to teaching and learning is based on the presumption that every experience has the potential to be an opportunity for learning. Learners are placed in an environment where they can assimilate information and develop skills by being personally involved. For HPE learners, experiential learning is likely to be work-based. This may be either in their own working environment or in a working environment that facilitates the learning of particular skills, for example dermatology out-patient clinic.

Adventure-based learning is also another form of experiential learning. Rohnke (1989) suggests that adventure learning may be used to illustrate a variety of theoretical concepts by use of specially designed outdoor experiences that can then be applied to a real world context. This can be particularly useful in areas such as team building or communication skills.

This list is by no means prescriptive or definitive. The challenge is to select the appropriate method of delivery for the subject matter and the audience. What works for one audience may not work for another. More traditional methods of delivery, such as lectures, seminars or workshops, may feel less taxing on educators' skills but they may be pleasantly surprised at the way an audience will respond to something new.

Summary

- The learning environment can influence the learning experience.
- Multidisciplinary learning can lead to more effective teamwork.

- Problem-based learning is a useful way of facilitating team learning.
- Distance learning is more effective if done within a support network.

References

Aronson E, Blaney N, Stephan C, Sikes J and Shapp M (1978) *The Jigsaw Classroom.* Sage, Beverley Hills, CA.

Barr H (2001) *Interprofessional Education 1997–2000: a review.* CAIPE, London.

Boud DJ (1985) Problem-based learning in perspective. In: D Boud (ed.) *Education for the Professions.* Higher Education Research & Development Society of Australia, Sydney.

Brockbank A (1994) Expectations of mentoring. *Training Officer* **30**, 86–88.

Burton J (2000) Multipractice and interprofessional learning in the community: a problem based approach to improving cancer care. *Education for General Practice* **11**, 51–57.

Candy P (1991) *Self-direction for Life Long Learning.* Jossey-Bass, San Francisco, CA.

Carruthers J (1993) In: B Caldwell and M Carter (eds) *The Return of the Mentor.* Falmer Press, London.

Chambers R, Wakely G, Iqbal Z and Field S (2002) *Prescription for Learning: techniques, games and activities.* Radcliffe Medical Press, Oxford.

Connor M, Byrne A, Redfern N, Pokora J and Clarke E (2000) Developing senior doctors as mentors: a form of continuing professional development. Report of initiative to develop a network of senior doctors as mentors 1994–1999. *Medical Education* **34**, 747–753.

Davis M and Harden R (1998) Problem based learning: a practical guide. AMEE Medical Education Guide No 15. *Medical Teacher* **21**, 130–140.

Department of Health (2001) *Working Together – Learning Together. A framework for lifelong learning.* DoH, London.

Downey P and O'Brien D (2001) Problem based learning: a valuable educational tool for use in the primary healthcare team and in training in general practice. In: S Field, B Strachan and G Evans (eds) *The General Practice Jigsaw.* Radcliffe Medical Press, Oxford.

Freeman R (1998) *Mentoring in General Practice.* Butterworth-Heinemann, Oxford.

Hartley S, Gill D, Walters K, Bryant P and Carter F (2001) Twelve tips for potential distance learners. *Medical Teacher* **23**, 12–15.

Mehrabian A and Ferris S (1967) Inferences of attitudes from non-verbal communication in two channels. *Journal of Counselling Psychology* **31**, 248–252.

Morton-Cooper A and Palmer A (1993) *Mentoring and Perceptorship.* Blackwell Science, Oxford.

Rohnke K (1989) *Cows Tails and Cobras II: a guide to games, initiatives, ropes, courses and adventure curriculum.* Kendall/Hunt Publishing Co, Iowa.

Ross N (1991) *Problem Based Learning in Undergraduate Medical Education: a discussion paper.* University of Birmingham.

Senge P (1990) *The Fifth Discipline.* Century Press, London.

Standing Committee on Postgraduate Medical and Dental Education (SCOPME) (1998) *Supporting Doctors and Dentists at Work – An Enquiry into Mentoring.* A SCOPME report. Standing Committee on Postgraduate Medical and Dental Education, London.

Watkins C and Whalley C (1993) *Mentoring Resources for School-based Development.* Longman, Harlow.

Wilkinson D (2000) *Turn on, Tune in, and Drop Out. Designing responsive learning environments.* Occasional paper for Oxford Learning and Teaching, Oxford.

9

Conclusions

We hope this book has emphasised four aspects of the thinking about HPE.

1 Those who administer or plan the delivery of medical education for GPs (at universities or postgraduate education departments) need to include HPE in their 'whole systems thinking'.
2 As a corollary to this systems approach, facilitators of HPE need to engage in 'joined-up thinking' with their neighbours in the continuum of GP education delivery. This includes trainers and course organisers of vocational training schemes, educational supervisors of enhanced registrars, and GP tutors for continuous medical education.
3 Thinking about HPE is to think about individual learners' needs and then to consider how they may best be addressed collectively. It is not about 'schemes' that consider collective needs and then try to tailor them to individuals.
4 HPE is new. Newness brings the chance to evolve and to demonstrate flexibility in development, but it also carries the responsibility to prove itself.

It is worth briefly revisiting these four essential aspects of HPE.

First, we showed how HPE is part of a continuum of education in general practice (*see* Chapter 1). The continuum is changing and HPE is also developing rapidly. The process of change must happen interactively as there is interdependence between the components of the GPs' education for independent practice (Figure 9.1).

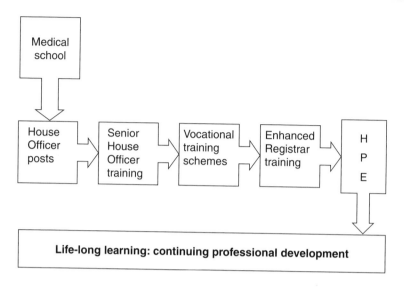

Figure 9.1: The interdependence between components of GPs' education for independent practice.

A little elementary systems thinking reveals two very important precepts.

1 GP education cannot and should not stand still.
2 Movement in one compartment has implications for all other compartments.

After all, compartmentalisation is only for administrative and budgetary convenience. In our NHS, the government pays for all components of doctors' education, from first setting foot in medical school to retiring from general practice.

Second, we have emphasised examples of joined-up thinking throughout this book. We looked at the research which showed what vocational training does well (*see* Chapter 1) and what gaps are left to fill (*see* Chapter 2). Research has shown that many learners new to independent practice recognise a need to learn more about aspects of practice management, something which trainers have previously struggled with, or thought they had covered adequately. Why don't we all put our heads together around curriculum planning? We need to recognise that learners learn best when the need to learn is evident (Ames, 1990) and perhaps we could encourage training practices to raise awareness of practice management issues but leave a lot of the detailed learning to be undertaken more effectively in the HPE years.

It makes educational sense, especially as there is widespread recognition that the vocational training scheme year has become overcrowded by the demands of summative assessment. But it takes us back to the systems thinking of our first point.

- If, in vocational training schemes, we place less emphasis on practice management, both COGPED and MRCGP will have to adjust the summative assessment framework.
- If learners are not to miss out on theses vital aspects of practice, HPE must attempt to reach all who enter independent practice. This means that the regulations must become more flexible in respect of career breaks.
- We must not lose one of the advantages of the teaching practices of vocational training schemes, which is that practice managers play an important part in the education of trainee registrars. These same practice managers must become involved with HPE.

The third point concerns individual learner-centricity of HPE. Having completed vocational training, learners who enter HPE have an informed awareness of the learning needs for general practice. HPE is therefore appropriately focused on the needs of the individual personal development plan (*see* Chapter 3). An analysis of educational needs is an essential tool, and we would like to see more GP trainers helping learners to develop their personal development plans before the end of vocational training, as this is an ideal time for an informed mentor to work on a one-to-one basis. HPE facilitators can then continue the process of addressing learners' needs.

The last point concerns the flexibility essential for a new educational programme if it is to meet learners' needs. Two examples will illustrate this well.

The first is enhanced registrar training. Registrars who have extended their training by six months in order to experience project development in general practice will have very different needs from those who come straight out of vocational training. Facilitators need to connect with these learners and plan how best to use HPE to take forward the learning of the fast-track shapers of general practice in the future.

Also, SHO training is currently being extended in the light of the government paper, *Unfinished Business* (Donaldson, 2002). This is having a major influence on the continuum of education, to which we refer above. By being nimbly adaptive, HPE facilitators can ensure that learning support is tailored to the altered learning needs of those who have spent longer in hospital posts or in early general practice training. This once more emphasises the need for 'whole systems thinking' and for personal development planning.

One of the shapers of modern medical education was Abraham Flexner. It was he who recognised that all learning was self-learning. Referring to medical students, he said, 'students learn more than they are taught'. The task for HPE is to enable the learning, which new practitioners will continue to develop throughout their careers.

References

Ames C (1990) Motivation: what teachers need to know. *Teachers College Record* **91**, 409–421.

Donaldson L (2002) *Unfinished Business: proposals for reform of the Senior House Officer grade*. DoH, London.

Index